OUT OF THE DARKNESS

I AM YOGA, JUST DO IT, DAMMIT!

AUDREY O'MARRA

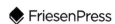

One Printers Way
Altona, MB R0G 0B0
Canada

www.friesenpress.com

Copyright © 2022 by Audrey O'Marra, CYA-E-RYT550
Kaitlin de Boer, Editor
Brandon Hoto, Editor
First Edition — 2022

All rights reserved.

No part of this publication may be reproduced in any form, or by any means, electronic or mechanical, including photocopying, recording, or any information browsing, storage, or retrieval system, without permission in writing from FriesenPress.

The content in this book is the author's experience of how Yoga has improved their wellbeing!
The author takes no responsibility for any practices mentioned in the book resulting in harm to the Reader.
This book details the author's personal experiences with and opinions about the practice of Yoga. The author is not a licensed healthcare provider. Statements in this text are not intended to diagnose, treat, cure, or prevent any condition or disease, nor intended as a substitute for consultation with a licensed healthcare professional.
Attributions for quotes and images herein are documented in Works Cited.

ISBN
978-1-03-911288-9 (Hardcover)
978-1-03-911287-2 (Paperback)
978-1-03-911289-6 (eBook)

1. Health & Fitness, Yoga

Distributed to the trade by The Ingram Book Company

Table of Contents

Prologue:
    A Journey out of the Darkness   v

I   **Misery in Life Is Inevitable**   1

II   **The Philosophy and Psychology of Yoga**   11

    Self-Study: Behind the Journey Within   11

III   **What Is Yoga?**   28

    A Journey Toward the Self   28

    The Main Types of Yoga   38

    The Five Types of Thought Waves (or Modifications of the Mind)   46

    The Eight Limbs of Yoga   50

| IV | **The Darkness** | **66** |

| V | **Where Your Journey Begins** | **80** |

In the words of Pema Chödrön,
"Start Where You Are" 80

| VI | **Returning to the Light** | **93** |

| VII | **My Sādhanā** | **98** |

Works Cited **105**

Prologue:

A Journey out of the Darkness

Even though the light is on,
The darkness is still there.
We must not run from the darkness.
We must walk with courage into it.
Walk softly into the darkness
And take the light with you.
The light exists within us all.
It is only degrees of light
That separate us from one another.
Life has a way of diminishing that light,
So come take a journey out of the darkness!

An Earth Angel is an individual who is on the planet to uplift and support others on this journey of life. My first thought was that it was going to be easy to narrow down my Earth Angels. While there are many that immediately come mind—those that uplifted me when I needed it and supported me when I was down—there are also many individuals who have challenged every ounce of my being, who have made my experience along the road of life rocky, painful, and downright hard. I appreciate those who made the journey easier, but I must acknowledge that it was the latter that lit a fire under my ass and kept me going. There's a part of my character that will dig deep and prove someone wrong when they tell me I can't do something.

If life is but the expression of the fears and desires we hold within ourselves, the manifest world is of our own creation. Our job on this planet is to clean up our own inner world of fears and unresolved issues. The people we meet each day serve us in one way or another, to either feed our fears or enrich our deepest desires. When I catch myself reacting to a situation, I remind myself that I am creating this, and this is an opportunity to wake up. I have learned that the people in our lives do not necessarily change when we wake up. Instead, our experiences with them change. The person you perceived as an enemy could now become your confidant. That job you hated now gives you a sense of fulfillment. When we begin to see everything as part of ourselves, we no longer feel separate from the world but instead experience a profound sense of belonging.

I deeply believe that it is my job to become an Earth Angel for those who come across my path, to uplift them whenever I can, to be kind, to forgive those who have trespassed against me, to love my neighbour as myself, and above all else, to love God with all my heart and soul.

> Promise Yourself
> To be so strong that nothing can disturb your peace of mind.
> To talk health, happiness, and prosperity to every person you meet.
> To make all your friends feel that there is something in them.
> To look at the sunny side of everything and make your optimism come true.
> To think only the best, to work only for the best, and to expect only the best.
> To be just as enthusiastic about the success of others as you are about your own.
> To forget the mistakes of the past and press on to the greater achievements of the future.

> To wear a cheerful countenance at all times and give every living creature you meet a smile.
> To give so much time to the improvement of yourself that you have no time to criticize others.
> To be too large for worry, too noble for anger, too strong for fear, and too happy to permit the presence of trouble.
> To think well of yourself and to proclaim this fact to the world, not in loud words but great deeds.
> To live in faith that the whole world is on your side so long as you are true to the best that is in you."[1]

I began writing this book in 2013, and as I write this section, it is now 2021. I'm in a very different place than I was when I began this journey of Yoga and the writing of this book. My goal is to finish this book before the end of 2021 and have it published. Otherwise … well, I'll have to change the date above. Thank you for coming along on this journey with me.

Life can be so terribly busy, and it seems to me that it just keeps getting busier every day. The connections we make on social media have made the world seem much smaller, and while it has its benefits of keeping us all connected, it also has downsides as well. We have all these forms of communication—texting, Facebook, Instagram, email, and WhatsApp, just to name a few—and holy crap, by the time you check and respond to all your messages, who has time to read a book, never mind write one? If you're currently reading this, that means I got it finished, so yay for me!

My purpose for writing this book is twofold: to share my story of getting out of the darkness I was once in, and to share with you the magic of my Yoga practice, which helped to transform my life. When I say "darkness," I'm referring to my emotional state of mind, my body's physical state, and my mental state.

---

[1] C.D. Larson, *Your Forces and How to Use Them* (Eastford, CT: Martino Fine Books, 2012), vi.

I was anxious and depressed, and I didn't take good care of myself. I had a lot of work ahead of me, but that wasn't the focus of my practice. Something hooked me on this practice of Yoga. The first time I lay down on my mat, I felt something—something real, something magic! When I use the word "magic," I don't mean that it was some esoteric experience, but it was an experience of just being still, listening to my breath, getting out of my head and into the present moment. My experience that first time in *Savasana*, or "corpse pose," has never left me; it was the first time in my life I felt the heaviness of life's burdens soften, if just for a few minutes.

For each of us, the experience of Yoga is something different, and that's OK. I simply wish for you to find that moment when life's heaviness softens in you as well. If you're reading this book, you've either tried Yoga or are about to. Whichever is the case, I'm grateful to be part of your journey. This journey can be rocky at times, but it's a journey worth taking, nonetheless. My deepest wish for you is that you get hooked on Yoga as well!

I've been practising Yoga since 2007, and every day my practice becomes deeper, along with my understanding of its benefits. Like the Bible states, "You will know them by their fruits" (Matthew 7:16a). The fruits of Yoga are plenty, but you need to practise it to reap the fruits it provides. Yoga is not a religion. Anyone, no matter your faith (or lack thereof), can practise it. Its roots, however, are steeped deeply in the Hindu practices of India. There's a spirituality and sensuality to Yoga; the word itself means to *Yuk*, or to unite body, mind, and spirit. By "spirit," I'm referring to that part of your being that enters your body when you're born and leaves when you take your last breath. What happens in between is life. Our society teaches us that happiness comes from things and circumstances, but Yoga teaches us that happiness comes from within ourselves. In Yoga, our individual Soul is referred to as *Atman*, and when we practice Yoga, the true goal is to Unite, or *Yuk* with the Divine, known in the Hindu tradition as *Brahman* and considered the highest universal principle.

Self-study is at the core of our Yoga practice. Looking within takes courage, and when we start to uncover the realms of the unconscious, it can be a bit scary to say the least. This self-study is the core of Yoga: even if the outer circumstances in our life aren't perfect, we learn to look at life differently. We no longer look outside of ourselves for validation, and our outer world starts to reflect our inner world. You have to appreciate the irony of this realization.

I mentioned that the practice of Yoga bears fruits. Essentially, what you put into your practice; you will get out of it. What are some of the fruits? To name a few, the practice of *asanas* brings strength and flexibility. The practice of *pranayama*, which is the practice of breath control, aids in calming and strengthening the nervous system and oxygenating the blood stream. It also prepares you for the practice of meditation, which has its own benefits. Those benefits will be discussed later in this book.

The name of the book may bring some frowns to many a seasoned Yogi, as non-harm is the first limb of Yoga. Some may be offended by the name, but it is meant to awaken, not to harm. Yoga is an Eastern practice, which means it's not based on a hamstring stretch. In the West, we are constantly bombarded with images of what appear to be perfect people doing perfect Yoga poses. This image, while seemingly beautiful, may give the individual the wrong idea of what Yoga truly is. It gives the impression that only seemingly perfect people can do Yoga. This is so far from the truth. No matter what your age, size, gender, physical condition, ethnicity, or social status, you *can* do Yoga. *The key is to do it, dammit!* There are so many different types of Yoga and different paths, but all lead to the same destination: to the true self!

The proverb "You can bring a horse to water, but you cannot make it drink" is so true. You can give people the tools to heal, but ultimately, it's everyone's personal choice whether they choose to use those tools. I use the term "heal" very loosely here as encompassing all the benefits Yoga has to offer an individual. We affect each other on subtle levels every day through our thoughts, intentions, and actions. Taking up a Yoga practice can bring you health and well-being, and the by-product of that practice can bring the same to others around you. I don't know about you, but I find that concept fascinating, and it leaves me with some sense of responsibility for the well-being of others. I am my brother's keeper. In a world that teaches the opposite, this is a concept you'll come to understand should you chose to take the Yoga journey.

You may not be able to touch your toes, but you can learn to breathe properly. You may not be able to stand on your head, but you may be able to stretch your arms overhead. You may not be able to hold the warrior pose for more than four breaths, but you can hold it for two.

There are many styles of Yoga, and one of them will surely meet your current needs.

My intention is to give you enough information in this book to deepen your current practice, and if you haven't taken up a practice, to inspire you to do so. So let us begin!

Come share my journey to the self!

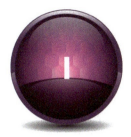

Misery in Life Is Inevitable

The human condition is one of misery and despair, just ask anyone. Are we ever happy? Are we ever satisfied with what we have? I challenge you to find a time in history when humans were content and living in harmony with one another. We seem to live in a state of constant misery, always looking at the proverbial glass as half empty. I seriously question anyone who says we see the glass half full. More often than not, this occurs on an unconscious level, below the surface of our awareness. Most people don't think, "Well, shit, I love misery!" But they say misery loves company, and how true is that? When we feel a sense of calm or a moment of happiness, we still sit in anticipation, waiting for the other shoe to drop, and inevitably it will!

I believe that the root of this misery is the fear of death. We do anything to avoid this truth. It's much easier to look outside of ourselves at the miserable world than it is to look inside and face our own fears. Life is about change. For everything there is a season. Our own emotional well-being can never come from an outside source; it must come from within. With the knowledge that this life is transient, we look at ourselves differently. We realize that our bodies are a vessel for our soul, and that these vessels will grow old and eventually die. Does that mean we cease to exist? I don't believe so. That wouldn't make any sense at all. I think of it like a receiver that picks up a radio station. The frequency of the station needs the radio to receive the signal, just as our soul needs a body to live in. The signal is still there, regardless of whether or not there's a radio to pick it up.

We say we want happiness, but look deep within yourself and ask just a few simple questions: What do you focus on? Usually, the negative. Any news station will confirm that. For every act of violence there's an act of kindness, but what do you suppose gets the most attention? Those sensational stories that get the most response from the viewer. Happiness doesn't sell and can't be marketed the way misery can, except perhaps on special occasions like Valentine's Day and Christmas Day. That rush of adrenaline, that surge of anger at the injustice we see in the world gives us a sense of power over others, thinking we're better than them, that we would never do such a thing. *Oh, how awful they are!* we think. Don't kid yourself: we all have angels and demons within us; it's just a matter of our life circumstances bringing them out or quieting them down. When we remove the veils of ignorance, or *avidya*, in Sanskrit, we soon discover that deep within us are the same demons we condemn in others—they may just not be as prominent. The practice of meditation helps us to peel off the layers of ignorance that separate us from other human beings. We soon realize that you and I are not so different. We may not be the same sex, same colour, the same age, etc., but underneath it all, we are the same.

Nothing in nature is permanent, so why do humans think they are exempt from the same laws that govern everything else in the universe? What comes from nature will return to nature. Ashes to ashes, dust to dust. This is a certainty, yet we go through life with some denial of the fact that we will pass on from this body we currently inhabit. I know I have certainly spent much time trying to pass the notion of death from my mind ... that is, until I had to face the reality with the loss of my parents and my granddaughter in the space of three years. We can bury our heads in the sand, but the reality of death we cannot escape. None of us gets out of this life alive.

The attachment to life, or the fear of death, is called *abhinivesa* in the Yoga tradition. In the Indian teachings, it's believed that the chanting of *om*. also spelled "Aum," which is thought to be the essence or sound of God the Creator, will eliminate this affliction of attachment to the body and the ego. This chanting is similar to the Christian singing of "Amen." Yoga also teaches us that our bodies are impermanent, but our souls are eternal. This gives us some comfort that this life is not lived in vain. Something happens on the mat, a connection to some inner knowing, that I believe exists in all of us. As Deepak Chopra suggests, the "Gap" is the space between thoughts, where we find the state of awareness.[2] In the silence of the Gap, that space between the breath, between the thoughts, we connect with that eternal part of our being. We experience becoming aware that we are not our bodies, and we are not the roles that we play out in this life. You can read these words, but until you sit in silence and experience this for yourself, my words will be just that: words. There's a knowledge that does not come from texts, from prayers, from teachers, from pastors, from priests, or from gurus but from our own experiences with these practices. And it was in these practices that I found peace.

I believe misery also comes from a state of not feeling good enough, forever feeling as though we are somehow broken in our human condition. I'm only lovable if I behave in a certain way, and if I fit into the criteria of "good." But who gets to measure that goodness? I believe that many religions are based primarily on a scale of right and wrong. But how can one judge by those standards? Furthermore, who are we to judge one another? Which of us will cast the first stone (John 8:7)? Is this not the message Jesus was trying to teach us? What makes one sin more wrong than another, and where do we begin to separate our standards of right and wrong? If a law is imposed making it legal to kill another person for stealing, does that make it OK to do so? Heinous crimes are committed every day around the world that are considered OK in the eyes of the law, many of them committed by our officials with the mindset that they are doing

---

[2] D. Chopra, "The Gap," *Deepak Chopra.* 18 October 2014. https://www.deepakchopra.com/articles/the-gap/

so for the greater good. Once again, who gets to choose the scale for right and wrong? If we can just take some time to pause and look within, we can tune into our internal compass that naturally tells us what is right and wrong, and we can shift from blaming others for our misery.

So often we blame others, don't we? But we always have a choice, and that's one scary concept. We can't control what goes on around us, but we *always* have a choice regarding how we react to any situation. This is the key to healing. In my experience, this implication really pisses a lot of people off, because for many people, everything is always someone else's fault. When we can consciously make choices and take full responsibility for them, then we begin to understand that we *do* create our own reality. Even if the choice is to stay in a job that you dislike, or in a relationship you know is unhealthy, it's your choice to do so. By doing so, you live with the consequences without blame or resentment. This is a huge step on the Yoga journey. I know what you're thinking: "Really? You have no idea what life is like for me, you can't tell me all of this is my fault!" The Yoga path demands that you not blame or point fingers at anyone, including yourself. On the contrary, it *does* demand that you take responsibility for your life as it is at this very moment and make the internal shift so that you can make an external shift to new attitudes and new behaviours.

The Christian religion reinforces this belief that someone else is always to blame. Satan is to blame for every sin committed by humanity. "The devil made me do it!" Holy crap, growing up I had this huge fear of the devil and thought that this evil force was just waiting in the darkness for me to let my guard down so it could sneak in and make me do things I wouldn't otherwise do. I feared looking under the bed or in the rear-view mirror for fear the devil was there waiting for me. I've since realized that the demons do not live under the bed. They live *within me*. I can't imagine something in the outside world that doesn't live within me first. Certainly there's evil in this world, but that evil is the absence of light and love, not the presence of Satan. Yoga is God, in the sense that the word "God" implies a creator, something greater than we are. Yoga is light, and we are created to shine, to give light and love to others. Fear creates darkness, and love is the absence of fear. But fear can crush love. How many times has your fear stopped you from doing the things you love? It's not our darkness that we truly fear—it's our light!

The practice of Yoga helps us understand that we are one with each other. If one of us is broken, then we all are. Throughout human history, many have come to bring this message, but something in us rejects it. The ego wants what it wants, often at the expense of another person's happiness. But what if we had a deeper understanding—that we can all find happiness and that there is enough for everyone? Call me an idealist—and that's OK. I've been called many things in this lifetime, but I believe that if we can practise self-love and self-care, there will be no need for competition. It would be replaced by the understanding that we are all in this together, and that we all breathe in the same air, drink the same water, and shit out of the same hole.

Once we find true understanding and compassion for ourselves and others, we no longer need to compete or put ourselves above or below others. The scale of right and wrong becomes more of a moral compass looking inwards. Does this mean we go through life disregarding our actions and how they affect others? Of course not! It means we begin to look within. We begin to do the hard work of self-study and self-reflection. When we no longer feel the need to point fingers at anyone else, we begin to understand that we must take responsibility for our own life and choices.

Once we become aware of our deepest fears and the source of our misery—death—we can then begin the journey to being happy! As we begin this journey, though, we soon realize that there might be a problem. It *is* human nature to want to be happy, isn't it? "Life, Liberty, and the Pursuit of Happiness" is stated in the United States Declaration of Independence, and it's what most people strive for, including us Canadians. The problem is, we often look for this happiness outside of ourselves. Looking for happiness outside of our own being will only bring pain and suffering; the world will disappoint us in one way or another. Even if we get the object of our desire, the feeling will eventually wear off, and then what? Discovering that happiness lies within is the most liberating feeling. But it also brings great responsibility. Once we realize that we create our own misery, we have to take full responsibility for what has happened in our lives, along with what is currently happening. If you stop what you're doing and take inventory of your life, what do you see? Are you happy? Do you feel content in your relationships? Do you enjoy your job? Taking the time to reflect or meditate on your current situation gives you the insight to make any necessary changes. We can go for long periods of time living our life unconsciously, just going through the motions. Even worse than that is going through life knowing that happiness comes from within but not having the courage to make the internal changes needed to benefit our well-being. Remember that the outside world only reflects our inner world. Cleaning up our inner environment will shift the outer one as well.

If you ask my children, they'll tell you how frustrating it was for them to hear me tell them time and time again to turn the other cheek. That's not easy to do, especially when the world teaches and reinforces the opposite. If someone injures you in some way, you want to strike back in kind. But what have you gained? My goodness, there are times when I really would like to slap the cheek of the person who I feel has injured me. My reality is subjective to my belief system and to my fears and desires. What injures me may not have been an intentional act from another. If I react in a negative manner and slap the other's cheek every time I feel offended, then I create a Karmic debt toward myself that *I* must pay back, not them. That means I am responsible, not them!

This doesn't mean that you allow people to walk all over you. Setting healthy boundaries is part of the Yoga journey as well. It teaches you to take a few breaths, look at the given situation from a different perspective, and then act or not act, whichever the case may be. Non-action creates Karma as well as action; it's our intention that matters most. At the very least, stepping back and taking a few deep breaths before you act allows you to make a conscious choice instead of the usual preconditioned response we so often fall back on. Our unconscious mind rules us, and Yoga allows us to bring the unconscious to light.

So how do we do that? How do we shed light on the unconscious mind? We self-study. *Svadhyaya* is a Sanskrit word that means "self-study" or "self-analysis." It's one of the most beautiful sounding words I've ever heard, and it's a key element of the Eight Limbs of the Yoga Path, better known as *Raja Yoga*. Bad habits are developed over a lifetime and passed down from our families. Those bad habits can be changed, and our unconscious programming can be reset, somewhat like the reformatting of a computer hard drive. Think of your mind as a computer that can be reprogrammed with new information. This understanding can make your progress less personal and more effective in doing what's necessary to develop new patterns and eliminate bad habits. Once we determine bad habits, then we can choose to replace them with good habits. Our habits become a choice instead of a preprogrammed response.

Creating a void without having something to fill that space back up would be fruitless, and that's where the seeds of Yoga come into play; we pluck out the bad seeds and replace them with good seeds! If nurtured, we know that those seeds have unlimited potential, and to me that is so exciting. Deepak Chopra states, "In every seed is the promise of thousands of forests."[3] This is true, but it only takes one match to destroy that forest. When these new seeds of Yoga are planted, they are fragile and must be nurtured in order to take root and produce that forest. If we want that forest to grow, we must give it the proper balance of light, water, nutrients, and, yes, even rest.

When we put our happiness in the hands of another person or thing and they don't fulfill our needs, we often give up. The path of Yoga is a deep journey toward understanding your deepest fears and how to bring your deepest desires to light. We try to fill our lives with things that we think will bring us happiness and fulfillment, and when they don't, we become discouraged. Sometimes we even feel great aversion and repulsion toward these things if we perceive them

---

[3] D. Chopra, D., *The Seven Spiritual Laws of Success,* (1994), 12, https://taxuna.files.wordpress.com/2015/11/deepak-chopra-the-7-laws-of-success.pdf

as having caused us pain. The body and mind don't give up the lower pleasures of life until they have tasted something better.[4] That "something better" is the benefits that come with continued practise of meditation and Yoga. Meditation has a positive effect on mind, body, and spirit. Among the physical effects of meditation are lowered blood pressure, clear thinking, better concentration, and an overall sense of well-being as we tap into the dormant resources of the mind.

Even though Yoga can be spiritual in nature, it also has scientific merit. *Science Daily* has stated that "past research using neuroimaging technology has shown that meditation techniques can promote significant changes in brain areas associated with concentration."[5] The practices of Yoga affect the limbic system, which in turn affects our emotional responses. This gives us more control over our emotions, enhances concentration, and improves memory, to name a few benefits. For people like myself who have had deep traumas—and let's face it, who hasn't? —these practices can be most beneficial in restoring a sense of well-being and calmness.

From a spiritual standpoint, there's only one way to reach the divine and that is to go within. When Jesus said, "the kingdom of heaven is at hand" (Matthew 3:2b), I don't think he was referring to some far-off place in the cosmos but to something much closer, much more attainable. The *Yoga Sūtras of Patañjali* state that "citta may be restrained by profound meditation upon God and total surrender to him."[6] In a nutshell, we need to surrender to something greater that we are.

I may be asking a lot of questions, but I desire for you to think. Use your mind and your inner wisdom to discern the truth, just like Jesus taught, "the truth shall make you free" (John 8:32b). If society is a reflection of us, it's up to us to

---

[4] J.S. Mill, *Utilitarianism,* (1863), https://www.utilitarianism.com/mill2.htm.

[5] University of North Carolina, Brief meditative exercise helps cognition, *Science Daily*, April 19, 2010, www.sciencedaily.com/releases/2010/04/100414184220.htm.

[6] B.K.S. Iyengar, "Light on the Yoga Sūtras of Patañjali, (1993), 78, https://docer.pl/doc/sxe8es0.

change ourselves first, and then the rest will naturally change with it.[7] The only way to make any permanent change is to bring awareness. Awareness means being present, letting go of the past and not focusing on the future. That's no easy task, since we're conditioned by our past, and our habits determine our future. We are the sum total of our past actions, thoughts, emotions, and experiences in this life—or, if you believe in reincarnation, all of our past lives. So how can we change this pattern? That's the million-dollar question!

A famous quote often attributed to Gandhi says: "Your beliefs become your thoughts, your thoughts become your words, your words become your actions, your actions become your habits, your habits become your values, and your values become your destiny." Where do those beliefs come from, and how can we change them? Or do we want to change them at all? Some come from our family history, our culture, and our education system, while others are encoded in our DNA—the classic nature versus nurture debate. As we learn, our cellular structure encodes that information, much like computer software stores information. I'm not a biologist, nor am I a scientist. The description above is my limited understanding of how the process of learning occurs. I challenge you to explore this topic and find out for yourself. Keep searching until you find the answers you're looking for. My goal is to break it down to a level that anyone can easily understand and put into practice. The above statement is my belief. If you make it yours without doing some investigating, or simply dismiss it as pure nonsense, it becomes fact without credibility, or it becomes nothing at all. My hope is that you explore, do some research, practise, and learn for yourself what is truth and what is nonsense.

Many practices can bring us to a state of stillness in which we can reach that attainable goal. As previously mentioned, *om* is the most sacred of all sacred words, and by chanting this sacred word, we can remove all obstacles that cause disturbances within the mind. Such a simple concept, but it must be practised

---

[7] J.C. Maxwell, The *Difference Maker* (New York, NY: HarperCollins, 2006), 9.

in order to reap its benefits, and therein lies the problem. I can't say how many times I've suggested to people that they can commit to such a practice to help them manage the stresses in their lives, and the first answer I hear from them is, "Oh, I'm far too busy to take time for that." In the words an old Buddhist saying, "You should sit in meditation for twenty minutes every day—unless you're too busy; then you should sit for an hour." In order to reap the benefits of Yoga, you must do the work. Just do it, dammit!

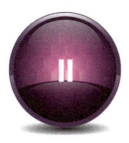

The Philosophy and Psychology of Yoga

Self-Study: Behind the Journey Within

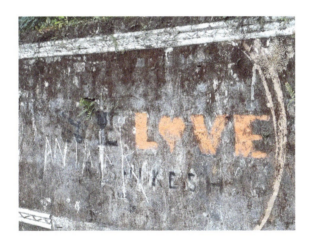

When you embark on a new journey of Yoga, there may be some concepts that seem strange to you. Beyond the physical discipline, the tradition of Yoga is steeped in mythology, symbolism, and philosophy. We will touch on some of these concepts, and the scope of this book will barely scratch the surface of other concepts.

What is Yoga? Well, if I had to define Yoga in one sentence, it would be: "Yoga is the study of self-reflection and self-care; a journey of the self through the self" (*Bhagavad Gita* 6:20). What benefit can there be in self-study? We can't change a displeasing habit without first becoming aware of it. There wasn't a magic cure to help me heal my suffering. It was the practice of self-study that gave me deep insight into my own demons. Shining the light helps us dissolve the darkness. I soon realized that I was the one creating most of the misery in my life. I had a big chip on my shoulder, and my actions and negative thought patterns only reinforced my misery. Self-study is one of the ongoing processes of our Yoga practice. Once we can recognize our own demons, we can make a conscious shift in our behaviour or, at the very least, acknowledge those demons. It could be as simple as recognizing that we gossip about others. We can then make the choice not to do that, or we can also choose to continue doing it. But it then becomes a conscious choice instead of a preconditioned behaviour. I'm drawn to the Eastern teachings because there is no blame, only cause and effect. Instead of getting trapped in a cycle of self-blame and self-sabotage, it becomes a matter of correcting negative thinking and negative actions that create a Karmic debt.

At times I struggle with the definition of Karma, especially when it comes to senseless acts of violence against seemingly innocent people. If every action has an opposite and equal reaction, how do we explain these acts of violence against the innocent? In general, I think the law of Karma makes perfect sense: what we reap we will sow. With this knowledge we understand that there are consequences for our actions, like gossiping about others. We then take full responsibility for our actions and the results that follow because of them. This is the law of Karma. It works with or without our awareness, so is it not better to be aware? Karma Yoga is seen at its finest in a life of service. Mahatma Gandhi exemplified the spirit of Karma Yoga: service and work without clinging to the fruits of action.[8] Tricky, isn't it? We work hard, we serve others, and of course we

---

[8] J. Hewitt, *The Complete Yoga Book*, (New York, NY: Schocken, 1990).

want some reward for our good deeds … no? By giving the fruits to God, living life in service—which is the core of Karma Yoga— you help maintain the world's welfare. By not being attached to the outcome, your actions serve the greater good rather than the illusion of the self. Krishna says, "He who is content in the Self, who is satisfied in the Self, who is pleased only in the Self: For him there is no need to act."

You will find on the journey of Yoga that there are many abstract teachings that can become confusing and be regarded as hocus pocus, to say the least. If you think of many of the concepts more as metaphors and apply the philosophies that we will explore in this text, you will gain more insight and deepen your own personal practice. During my meditation training, my dad would always ask me, "Which flavour of Kool-Aid are you drinking today?" He was referring to the Jonestown mass suicide, and how people can be brainwashed into doing just about anything, including taking their own life and the lives of others, according to their beliefs. Many religious followings have a deep history of violence, all in the name of "God." The Salem Witch Trials in the late 1600s to the more recent events of 9/11 are just two examples of this. People will go to great lengths to enforce their beliefs on others and punish those who don't comply. Some may argue that if we were to get rid of all religions, we would solve the problem of violence in our world, but I disagree! It's not religion that sparks hatred but fear of the lack of control over our own lives. It's intolerance of and a lack of respect for others that are at the root of it. It's the fear that "they" will change our way of thinking and living, threaten what we know to be true, and threaten our comfort zone. That comfort zone is, of course, an illusion.

Our Yoga practice helps us to remove the veils of ignorance that cloud us from the realization that we are light, we are meant to shine, we are born to live and love to the fullest of our potential as beings in a human body. We live on a planet that could be struck by an asteroid, see a dormant volcano explode, or experience some event that blocks the sun's light and ends life as we know it on the planet. The threat of massive world wars is always present, but still, we build this false sense of security. All of society, including culture, is built upon this illusion. And what is worse, we fool ourselves into thinking that security is obtainable. I guess this security helps us sleep at night. I lost endless nights of sleep trying to reconcile in my mind most of what I'd been taught about life and death. We're trained from an early age to believe this illusion: go to school, get good grades, get a good job, save until retirement, retire on a desert island with the sun beaming down on us ... blah, blah, blah. Seriously, this is a tragedy. In the meantime, we miss life while planning for a future that may never happen.

At first this may sound very discouraging, but the opposite is true. Once we come to the realization that: a) yes, we will die, and b) yes, there's always a chance that some disaster beyond our control may threaten and destroy our way of life, we will feel a freedom in breaking this illusion. Tim McGraw's song "Live Like You Were Dying" says it all. The lyrics remind us that we can't wait until tomorrow to live, but that we must live for today, and that fearing to live fully isn't living at all.

If you've spent any amount of time with someone who is facing death, you know that in their final moments, they see everything through a different lens. Take the time to smell the roses, to look at that beautiful blue sky, to breathe, love, dance, paint, make love, sing, go skinny dipping—and don't put all of your stock in some future that doesn't exist yet. We don't want to be reckless, but we *do* want to live in the moment and enjoy life rather than blindly going through the motions of existence so we can enjoy life twenty years from now. Life is now, in this very moment! Life is the most fragile and precious gift, so it should be cherished like the priceless jewel it is, and that jewel should shine brightly. To conclude, when we fear death and forget that we are an eternal being, we cannot truly live!

How do we begin this self-study? We begin with our thoughts. If we really take stock of our thoughts and emotions, we may notice that in our personal relationships we focus on the negative in others: What they said or didn't say that may have hurt us. What they did or didn't do to meet our expectations. We put so much of our happiness (or lack thereof) in the hands of others, when in reality it only exists within us. We create our own reality by our projections and judgements, which leaves us with a great deal of responsibility. It's much easier to just carry on and blame others.

We are the sum total of all our past actions, not only in this life but in our past lives. Whether or not you believe in reincarnation, we have the past lives of generations that have gone before us ingrained into our DNA. We're born into a certain social status, and breaking free of that status, or "Karma," takes a great deal of effort and self-awareness. Otherwise, no genetic imprint is changed, and the cycle will go on to become status quo. The sins of the father/mother become the sins of the sons/daughters for seven generations forward. I remember one specific event that happened just after I left high school. I had returned to the school one day to pick up one of my younger siblings, and the person I was with later mentioned that their friend had asked them what they were doing with me. We all make assumptions based on appearance, family names, and social status, whether we care to admit it or not. I remember feeling shame and confusion when this person told me what had been said. I just thought I was me. At that time, I didn't know I came with a label that said, "damaged goods." The sad reality was that I *was* damaged, very much so, and it would take me many decades to undo that damage and repair those shattered parts of myself. Before that realization, I would unfortunately add to my Karmic debt by continuing to make bad choices. Once I became aware that my choices were affecting my life negatively, I chose differently.

Once we have the courage to practise self-reflection, we can make any necessary changes in our character that can benefit not just our lives but the lives of our fellow human beings. Of all the philosophies of Yoga that we will practise, Karma is the most important to understand. Once we grasp its concepts, we can make positive changes to our already accumulated Karmic debt. Like gravity, the law exists regardless of our awareness of it.

Karma Yoga is the Yoga of action: "One cannot achieve freedom from karmic reactions by merely abstaining from work, nor can one attain perfection of knowledge by mere physical renunciation" (*Bhagavad Gita* 3:4). The "action" referred to in Karma Yoga differs from what we would commonly associate with action in our modern world. We're taught from an early age that to achieve prosperity, we must work hard, go to school, get good grades, get a good job, earn lots of money, etc. Things are always attached to the outcome. Karma Yoga focuses on doing those same actions in service of a higher good rather than being attached to the outcome. This is hard for us to wrap our heads around, as we're programed to only do good if we're rewarded for that good. We find it extremely hard to do good when there's no reward. But what if we could realize that we should do good *just for the sake of doing good*? Imagine the change we could make in the world! But there's a part of us that resists such thoughts, no? What reward is there for me if I get nothing in return?

By taking all our actions and doing them as if God were the one doing them, we detach ourselves from the outcome, and we don't create any more negative Karma. There's some overlap here, as with many other paths of Yoga, which we'll explore later. There's a great deal of overlap with Bhakti Yoga in particular, where God is the centre of focus in practice on and off the mat.

We can't avoid actions in our daily life; everything we do requires us to participate in life. Even non-action creates a Karmic ash. We can't avoid the outcome of Karma by not acting, and no debt goes unpaid. Eating, sleeping, working … whatever the case may be, we must act or cease to exist. "Therefore, giving up attachment, perform actions as a matter of duty, for by working without being attached to the fruits, one attains the Supreme" (*Bhagavad Gita* 3:19).

We carry out hundreds of tasks every day, some of which we really dislike. If I feel frustrated every time I do my dishes, or fold a load of laundry, I create energy that goes out to the universe only to return to me as an echo. The universe doesn't discriminate, and it doesn't know the difference between right or wrong; it only knows energy and information. What we give out we get back in the same manner. The emotions we carry within us are sent out like a beacon, and that same signal comes back to us like a boomerang. Many people struggle with making the same mistakes over and over again, and the result is always the same. Nothing changes unless something changes, and that change begins with working on your emotions and understanding what signal we are sending out to the world around us. Becoming aware is the first step to healing and changing our Karmic debt. I don't know about you, but I need examples for my mind to absorb these teachings.

If, for example I want love, but I haven't resolved my feelings of unworthiness, I'll continue to attract situations and people who validate the feeling of unworthiness in me. For me to make a shift, I have to do some self-study in order to uncover why I feel I'm not worthy, and for the most part this takes place on a subconscious level. That's why we focus on *feeling* during our Yoga practice; we feel whatever is happening in our bodies, our emotions, our thoughts. Once we do that, we can do the hard work of inquiry and uproot the false beliefs of our unworthiness. For me, it could have been something as simple as a caregiver shunning me as a child for not living up to their expectations. Love is earned and not freely given, right?

For you, it could be something completely different, but in the end, the feelings are the same. Once we can make the shift to practise self-love and self-acceptance, others' expectations of us aren't our concern any longer. We begin to realize that everyone is seeking love and acceptance, and that they project their lack of these onto us, as we do to them. It makes it much less personal. But these can be painful lessons to learn, and looking deep within takes courage, as you may be discovering.

When I was seven, my siblings and I moved into a house in Hamilton with my mom and our soon-to-be dad (and his children, our soon-to-be siblings) after being in and out of foster care for years. Soon after moving in, I made a friend, and her family took me for a day to go swimming at the bay just a few blocks from our house. It was such a fun day! I can still see the water, smell the breeze, feel the warmth on my face. Her family was welcoming and warm as well; it felt good and safe. I was full of sunshine and joy, only to return to a home full of anger and resentment. My dad was waiting for me at the door. He grabbed me and spanked me for being late. I was confused and terrified at the same time; my joy was stolen in that moment of his anger. I was seven years old. How was I to be responsible for being late? This fear became the basis of my existence, and still today with all of my progress, there's this underlying unsettling feeling that "If you have fun, Audrey, you will be punished!"

I'm not alone in these experiences, as many of us can tell the same stories. And back in the day, what we not call abuse was acceptable parenting. I've been reading a book recently called *My Secret Sister*.[9] It's a story of twins separated at birth; one is raised by her biological family, and the other is adopted out. The sister adopted out lived a life of love and trust, while the other a life of abuse and mistrust. When we are children, our happiness depends on our parents or care givers approval, as does our misery. I don't tell this story to shame my parents, because believe me, I have done some things as a parent I am certainly not proud of. When we know better, we have to do better.

Imagine you have an exam in the morning. You've studied as best you can, but all you can think about is you don't have clean clothes to wear to school, and you don't even have a toothbrush. There were 7 children and two adults, and going to the laundry mat was not cheap, nor was clothing all of us. So, you go to school wearing dirty clothes and brushed your teeth with your finger. Not only do you need to pass this test, but you also must "fit" into this mold society has crafted for a twelve-year-old and reach all the "markers" to progress to the next grade. You know the adults can't get their shit together, but they put an enormous amount of pressure on you to do just that, because that's the mandate set out by society and the education system. Again, all you can think about is that ham sandwich your classmate threw out at lunch time, right before they ate their snack pack. Who throws out a ham sandwich? I would trade my peanut butter sandwich for that ham sandwich, if I even brought my lunch that day! Most days, I felt embarrassed to even bring that peanut butter sandwich. And guess what, I sent peanut butter sandwiches to school with my children, because like my parents, that was what was cheap and what we could afford.

---

[9] H. Edwards, and J.L. Smith, J.L., *My Secret Sister.* (New York, NY: Pan Macmillan, 2013).

And now ... holy fuck! You have this damn test! If you don't pass, you face the scorn of the teacher for not studying hard enough: "You must try harder, Audrey!" You hear the teacher saying and as you listen to your parents argue about, it's all you can do to hold your sanity together and get through the night, let alone study. Yet this becomes the norm, and for the most part, you don't question any of it. You begin the process of self-loathing. The fear of your parents finding out you have failed settles in.

The part of you that I call the "shitty committee" is well-established: "you" are the failure, not the dysfunction of the world you're living in. "Study harder," "Be better," "Don't be so fat," "Children should be seen and not heard," "You're the smart one," "I'm so disappointed in you," "Try harder, try harder, try harder."

Something in you knows this is so wrong, but you have no control. You just do the best you can to get through today. And the next day. And the next day. Soon these days turn into all of your life: well-established yet completely fucked up and built upon quicksand. You want to scream, but those screams are silenced. They become internalized until they reach a point where "you" no longer exist. No one will listen. No one truly gives a damn. They know, they *all* know about the constant abuse, but no one wants to step in. So you stuff it down, and as you grow into adulthood, it grows within you until you've also convinced yourself that this life you're living is "normal." Still believing that "you" are to blame, you continue to make choices based on this belief.

And then you hit the wall—that place in the psyche where you realize that if you don't turn back, you won't come back at all. You'll die if you don't turn this shit around. You may be alive in body, but your soul is damaged. It ... no, *you* ... need to express all these feelings. This reality you're currently living is not what your soul has in mind. This is the point where I think many choose suicide. They check out; the crack is too big to make it back across. Yoga helped me dust off the old furniture and build the bridge back across on a much stronger foundation. I've learned on this healing journey that it's crucial to have the courage to be vulnerable and ask for help when you need it. If you don't get the help you need at first, keep asking. There are so many amazing Yoga teachers and spiritual healers out there. Just keep searching until you find the one that can guide you to your own ability to heal.

Yoga can do the same for you!

The next step is to actually apply these teachings to your practice. Please, I want you to understand that I don't blame my parents—well, maybe a small part of me still holds a deep resentment toward my biological father for discarding us like garbage and leaving my mom alone with five small children, but I digress. I have great respect and reverence for the parents that raised me and worked very hard every day to provide a home as best they knew how. I have been practising and studying Yoga for decades now, and it has healed so many wounds I thought would never heal. You may wonder why I would share my personal stories. Well, it takes courage to look at our scars, and when we can do that, others find the courage to do the same. When we speak our truth about our own experience, others also find the courage to do so. Only in darkness can evil hide, it cannot hide in the light! Speaking out helps shine light on that darkness, and this is what this book is all about.

I have been struggling with deleting content of my story, as not to upset people, but I remind myself that this is my story, my experience of my life. There is no judgement in anything I share, for each of us has our own truth, and our own experience, and what is significant for me, may not be for someone else who shared a similar upbringing. And many times, then not, children, heck even adults don't speak out because they feel somehow, they are to blame. They don't want their parents angry with them, they don't want others realities shattered, so they stay silent, and it was in silence I was dying inside.

This is such a hard thing to recover from, but I honestly believe that if you can learn to love yourself, you can heal your inner child. What was most effective for me was making a commitment to my own well-being and putting myself first. I had to deeply examine the pattern I was currently caught up in, and then I had to change it. I made a commitment to that inner child to look after her, to keep her safe so that she could enjoy life without constant fear and a need for approval from others. As an adult, I have a choice—even if those choices are limited, and most times they are—to make that commitment to myself.

This is my challenge to you, my reader: make the same commitment to yourself. Your life may be different from mine, but it is *yours* to work with, *and you ARE worth this work!* If you think you're being selfish in making this choice, please remember that when you find happiness within, it is so much easier to allow others around you the same privilege. When you no longer allow others to have a negative effect on you, you no longer put the pressure of your happiness on another.

If I go to work every day with the notion that my co-workers are the cause of my unhappiness, I'll likely project that onto them, and my reality will mirror that misery back to me. On the other hand, if I go to my job every day with a positive attitude and respect for my co-workers, I'll project a completely different energy. Most of the time we do this on an unconscious level, but once we're aware of what we're doing, we have the power to choose how we act toward others. Does that mean that our co-workers will never do anything to annoy us? Of course not! It means that we'll react to it differently. When we realize that they have the same fears and desires we have, we can look at the situation from a different perspective, and in doing so, we can change our reaction to the situation. The most difficult thing to realize is that they are not aware, and that leaves them at a disadvantage. Once we become aware, that leaves us with a deeper sense of responsibility. I have struggled with this concept. Surely I am not responsible for others' bad behaviour, especially when it affects me. I have no control over them, but I can learn to control my reaction to any particular situation. I can choose to just walk away and turn the other cheek (Matthew 5:38–42), or I can retaliate in kind and keep the never-ending cycle of suffering going. There is freedom in the knowledge that their ignorance of their behaviour does not exempt them from the bad fruits it will yield, nor are those fruits my burden to carry.

While actions speak louder than words, our intentions speak even louder. If I hold the door open for someone with a smile on my face, it may appear that I'm acting out of kindness. But if my thoughts and feelings don't match the act, the act is done in vain. If I hold the door open for someone, it should be with feelings of kindness and humility. We should do our duty for duty's sake, as taught in the *Bhagavad-Gita.* The *Gita* is a religious text considered to be the sacred "song of God." While it's based in Hinduism, its message is universal. It is said to have been composed in about 200 BC, and it contains a discussion between the deity Krishna and the Indian hero Arjuna on the nature and purpose of life. Arjuna asks Krishna, "Then by what is a man compelled to commit evil, *varshneya*, seemingly against his own will, as if urged thereunto by force?" (3:36). Krishna tells Arjuna that it is not the action that causes the result but the desire, the anger, and the veils that keep us from our true nature. By controlling our senses, or *Gunas,* and not being attached to the outcome, we prevail. "Above the body are the senses; Above the senses is the mind; Above the mind is intellect; Above the intellect: the self" (3:42). So even with the best of intentions, I must remember that holding the door open should not be attached to any certain outcome. For example, the next time someone fails to open the door for me, I shouldn't think, *Well, I held the door open for so-and-so, so I expect the same thing in return.* Sadly, I see this attitude even in the Yoga community, even among those with the awareness that we are human and fall into old thinking patterns very quickly.

    The concept of non-attachment to an outcome is hard for our Western society to comprehend, let alone practise. We think that the fruits we've worked for should be ours and ours alone, but this serves no good in the end. For what good are my fruits if my neighbour is starving (3:17)? In other words, there's no need to hold the door open if the end result is merely to serve the self.

    My parents worked hard labour jobs their entire lives, only to retire and die within two years from cancer. Their belongings were pillaged through and sold for a small fraction of their worth … at least, the worth of what a lifetime of hard work should have given them. It was very painful to watch this process—an entire lifetime reduced to some boxes being sold at an auction. Through this process, I learned a valuable lesson: everything is impermanent, and it's an illusion to think otherwise. If you look around the room you're currently sitting in, consider that in a thousand years, none of those items will be there, including you. So why on God's green Earth do we strive for possessions that in the end hold no real value?

When I think about the hard work my parents did to acquire those possessions, I realize that they wore out their bodies as well as their minds. They both came from poverty and made a vow not to follow in the footsteps of their parents. Of course we want nice things, and we want to live in comfort. It's the attachment to our possessions, the keeping up with the Joneses, that causes us suffering. As soon as we acquire something new, it loses its lustre. We are a throwaway society: when something breaks or wears out, in the trash it goes. The Japanese use a technique known as *Kintsugi* to repair broken china and pottery. They take lacquer mixed with gold or silver to fill in the cracks. What a beautiful concept! Couldn't we apply that same technique metaphorically to all areas of our lives?

In our Western culture, we're raised to believe that by our works, we gain results. If we work hard, we'll move ahead in life and attain the things we believe can make us happy. We go to school to learn and obtain jobs that will pay us enough to live comfortably, with nice homes and nice cars. Krishna warns about serving only the self and teaches that humans are to perform their duty while remaining unattached to the fruits of that work—not to go about trying to convince others of the proper way to act, but to set the bar high and be an example for others to follow. Krishna says, "Whatever the best of men does—This and that—thus other men do; Whate'er the standard that he sets—That is what the world shall follow" (3:21).

Our minds are immensely powerful things, and they've been programmed over the years to react to situations based on our past experiences and our biological makeup. Karma is likewise an immensely powerful force but one that we can work with once we become aware of how it operates. Changing our Karmic pattern is no easy task; emotions like jealousy, anger, and frustration are powerful. When they're triggered, we react accordingly and in turn build upon our

Karmic debt. Again, it's the attachment to things that causes us the most suffering. We're attached to our belongings, our loved ones, our jobs, and so on, and when they're taken away from us, or they don't meet our expectations, we suffer. Does that mean that we don't acquire any belonging or form any relationships? Do we act in the extreme and become monks and swear off worldly possessions altogether? I don't believe so. I think it means that we cherish what we have with the knowledge that all will eventually pass away.

We can't escape the trials and tribulations life will hand out. We are born; therefore, we will die. That is certain. What we do with the time we're given in between is the true key to happiness and contentment. It seems a bit gloomy to say the least, but it also leaves us with a great opportunity to *really* live life with all of its ups and downs and many layers. The Buddha says that suffering in this life is inevitable,[10] and until we fully embrace that, we can't find true happiness. This seems contradictory, but it's the only true way to contentment. The Buddha says, "Suffering, pain, and misery exist in life; Suffering arises from attachment to desires; Suffering ceases when attachment to desire ceases."[11] It's as simple as that!

Raja is a Sanskrit word that refers to one of the three energies that the universe and everything in it is made of. According to teachings of Yoga, the universe is comprised of three basic energies, known as the *Gunas*.

1: *Tamas:* sluggish or dull energy.
2: *Sattva*: pure, light, calm energy; and

---

[10] The Buddha is often misquoted as using a more nihilistic phrase that simply states, "Life is suffering," which suggests that to be alive is to suffer, or that the purpose of life is to suffer. More accurately, Buddha simply acknowledges that life will inevitably include suffering in some form, and the acceptance of this fact is an important step in achieving happiness and fulfillment.

[11] R. Kurtus, "Four Noble Truths of Buddhism," School for Champions, October 6, 2018, https://www.school-for-champions.com/religion/buddhism_four_noble_truths.htm#.YRA0QIhKiM9

3: *Raja*: restless, passionate energy that can be thrown out of balance by our desires.

When this energy is in balance, it can be used as fuel to better one's life and the lives of others. But when out of control, this energy can consume and destroy. We can take the energy of our suffering, cultivate it, and keep the fires burning at a steady pace instead of letting the fire burn out of control. For example, if I feel offended by something someone has done to me, I will feel some sort of suffering, usually some frustration and a desire to attack. Instead of allowing the fire of anger to rage inside of me and spill out onto the person I think offended me, I can make a conscious choice to feel the frustration and anger without retaliation. I can try and look past the perceived offence, or I can remove myself from the situation. Every one of us has our own story and, therefore, our own demons!

One might think, *I have a wife, but look over there ... what a beauty! If only I could have that woman, I would truly be happy. I have a house, but look over there ... what a beauty! If I could only have that house, I would truly be happy. I have food in my new refrigerator, but look at that steak. If I could only afford that, I could truly be happy. If I could only find the answers to life's most perplexing questions, that would surely bring me true happiness. That church looks wonderful. I wonder if I could find happiness and the God I seek there?* More questions. I ask you to please take a moment to reflect on your thoughts and desires. Do you feel satisfied with your life, or are you always looking for the next thing to bring you gratification, which will fade as soon as you acquire it?

Modern science explores all the mysteries of the universe and only comes up with new and more complex questions. In our day and age, it holds the monopoly on life and its mysteries, and anyone seeking wisdom outside of modern science is, for the most part, considered "ignorant." *Avidya* is a Sanskrit word that means "ignorance" or, more accurately, "mistaking the unreal for the real" and being attached to what is impermanent. All under the sun and moon will pass away. So why do we spend so much time during our short trip here on

Earth longing for something we may never have, while missing the pure beauty of what we *do* have? We live in a society that constantly reinforces that longing: new this, new that, always looking to the horizon for that next fix. While these things do bring us temporary joy, we will eventually get bored and move on to the next new gadget.

The place I seek is and always has been within me, as it is in you. My searching has led me back home to me, for all the answers to the mysteries of life exist within. All I had to do was slow down enough to hear the answers. While reading scriptures and spiritual texts is important and will help us along our journey, our true knowledge is innate. All those scriptures point us in that direction. For example: "seek, and ye shall find" (Matthew 7:7, KJV).

The root of Yoga is to still the restless chatter of the mind long enough to hear that small voice within. That voice, I believe, is the voice of God. Which God you hear is a personal choice. Your upbringing or where you were born will determine what God, if any, you worship. To me, there is only one, but there are many ways to reach him or her. Many wars have been fought on this planet to determine which God is the "right" one. Being raised in the belief that Jesus was and is the only true salvation has left me with some lingering doubts as to what the true path is. I'm no expert on religion, and I certainly have my doubts about the afterlife. I do believe with all of my heart that there is an intelligent being that created this universe and everything in it. I also believe that this intelligent being sends us messengers—like Jesus, Patañjali, and the Buddha, to name a few—to show us how to navigate this life on Earth. Those enlightened beings understood what it is like to be human as well as divine. I'm not a scholar of religion, nor do I pretend to be. I think that any religious text can be twisted and interpreted in many ways. It's the twists that cause separation between you and I, and when your way of thinking threatens my way of thinking, that creates the urge for me to convince you to think my way. The teachings of Yoga urge the opposite: they ask me to look within at the barriers that stop me from seeing your point of view. Accepting our differences allows us both to live in a manner that gives each of us the space to be ourselves.

On this journey of life, I have discovered that true happiness lies in the ability to be oneself, but whatever that will be is specific to each individual. "... the truth shall make you free" (John 8:32b) doesn't mean to confess all your sins to be free ... although confessing a sin does make one feel better. In this context, I believe it means being true to oneself. *Satya* is a Sanskrit word that means "truthfulness" and reaffirms that being truthful means living a life without bringing harm to others. One of the Reiki principles is to live your life honestly. As Virginia Wolfe famously wrote: "If you do not tell the truth about yourself, you cannot tell it about other people."[12] Our truth gets strangled over time by others' expectations, our roles in our family, and our roles in society. If we don't "fit" we somehow feel like we've not only failed ourselves but also others. Looking within helps us find our truth and live a life that's authentic to who we are. When we can do that, we are free!

If I live my life according to what I think others want from me, I am in no way being truthful. I will eventually become resentful of them and myself for not following my own potential as a human soul on this planet. If a rose seeks to become a daisy, it will wither and die. No amount of seeking will take away the fact that it is a rose. If God created us in his or her image, we were created perfectly just the way we are, with all of our layers and complexities. With that in mind, I don't feel the burden of "sin" in the context that is taught in many religious institutions. I do, however, come to the knowledge that every action does have an equal and opposite reaction. So the choices I make determine my destiny. With that knowledge, I can mold my life accordingly.

The big question is, "What is my truth and where is this happiness I seek?"

In asking this question, my journey began!

---

[12] V. Woolf, V., *The Moment and Other Essays*, 1947, Project Gutenberg Australia. http://gutenberg.net.au/ebooks15/1500221h.html.

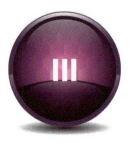

What Is Yoga?

A Journey Toward the Self

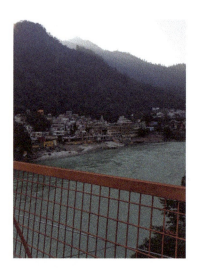

Who am I? Where did I come from? Where am I going? Why was I born? What happens when we die? No matter what faith or social group you fit into, at one point or another in our lives we all question our very existence. Is there a God? If there is, why does he or she not show him or herself to us? This "Christ" who was born some two thousand years ago, whose second coming has been foretold ... where is he? If he died for my sins, then does that mean I can go about sinning without any fear of my soul being in danger? With so many questions, how do we find the answers to them? "Seek and ye shall find" (Matthew 7:7, KJV). This verse has always stuck with me. While I can't tell you that I've found the answers to all of these questions, I can tell you with certainty I have found some resolve with them. I didn't find the resolve from reading sacred texts, attending church on a regular basis, or from years of service to others. I found this resolve by sitting quietly on my mat in meditation. There is a stillness within that is beyond words, beyond any description. The aim of all Yoga practice is to attain the truth wherein the individual soul identifies itself with the supreme soul, or God. I had finally found my truth!

The practice of Yoga is the journey of the self, through the self. The journey to the divine within, to the source of all creation. Some people use the term "universe." I use the term "God." Everything starts from within; I believe we are born with the knowledge of God already wired in our DNA. If you think about it rationally, why wouldn't we be? Aren't we always on a search to prove God does or doesn't exist? Why would you go on a quest to prove that something doesn't exist unless you believe on some level that it does? While some may ask these questions, they may never take the time to do the self-analysis necessary to find the answers. Our world has an abundance of information literally at our fingertips. External knowledge is not enough; it doesn't fulfill our soul, and all that external information doesn't prove or disprove the existence of something greater than ourselves. That knowledge can only come from within. It can only be experienced; it can only be revealed.

According to the Patañjali Sūtras there are three categories of valid knowledge: perception, inference, and scriptural or revealed authority.[13] We experi-

---

[13] P.R. Tigunait, (2021). Yoga Sūtra 1.6-1.7 Translation and Commentary. *Yoga International.* https://yogainternational.com/article/view/yoga-sutra-1-6-1-7-translation-and-commentary

ence direct perception during meditation; I searched for many years outside of myself for the answers to all of the above questions. It wasn't until I sat quietly in meditation that I finally found the peace I was seeking and the silent answers to the questions that stirred my soul. In order to *experience* God, it must be revealed to us, and it is my strong belief that it comes in the silence of the Gap. As mentioned in the previous chapter, Deepak Chopra suggests that the Gap is the space between thoughts, where we find the state of awareness.[14] The idea of the Gap has been elaborated upon in his blog,[15] including how one can make spiritual progress within this state of awareness.[16]

Recall my personal definition of Yoga earlier in this book: "Yoga is the journey of the self, through the self, to the self." We may have book knowledge, but without the practical application, it's just knowledge. I can read a recipe in a book, but until I have the ingredients and follow the directions as set out in the recipe, it's just words in a book. Reading about how to make chocolate chip cookies is definitely not the same thing as actually making them, and once they are made, you get to eat them. The "fruit" of baking the cookies is the pleasure you receive from eating the tasty morsels, if you followed the recipe correctly.

It's the same with our Yoga practice. Reading ancient texts and looking at beautiful videos of Yoga routines will not bear the "fruits" of Yoga. Only by applying the techniques with effort and determination will you see the "fruits" of your practice.

I continue to meet people who seem lost, searching desperately for relief from their physical and emotional pain. They'll try anything to dull that pain, and there's certainly no shortage of ways to do so. Drugs, alcohol, sex, food,

---

[14] Chopra, D. (2014). The Gap. *Deepak Chopra.* 18 October 2014. https://www.deepakchopra.com/articles/the-gap/

[15] Ibid.

[16] Chopra, D. (2020). Progress in the Gap. *Deepak Chopra.* 12 May 2020. https://www.deepakchopra.com/articles/progress-in-the-gap/

sports, work, shopping, and even the spiritual journey can become an escape. The problem with these fixes is that they're short lived, and the next fix needs to be stronger in order to dull the pain. Prior to my Yoga journey, I was one of those people who needed to escape my internal pain, and some days I feel I still am. At the point where I started my Yoga journey, I had a victim mindset. While our past has a significant impact on our current behaviour, the *choice* to change my preconditioned responses was mine. I believe that my *choices* alone will determine the fate of my soul, and I believe Jesus was the ultimate Yogi. His teachings were very specific as to how we are to conduct ourselves on the Yoga and life journey: non-harm, truthfulness, living a life for God, turning the other cheek, and loving your neighbour as you would love yourself. In order to love your neighbour, you need to learn to love yourself first. I had to learn to let go of the pain of the past and love myself—not an easy task when you have a lifetime's worth of negative voices in your head telling you otherwise.

Do we ever find the answers to life's most perplexing questions? You'll have to determine for yourself, as it's your responsibility to seek out the answers to these questions. It's my pleasure to be on this journey with you as you seek them out. The practice of Yoga is one of self-study, to unite, or *yuk*, all parts of self. When I began my journey of Yoga, the parts of myself were very scattered. There are days when I still feel a bit scattered, and when I do, I go to the mat! The practice of Yoga is my refuge, my sanctuary, my sacred ground where I connect with my higher self. It takes me into the present moment, out of my head, and away from life's responsibilities, if only for a brief time. This time on the mat allows me to ground myself and find that stillness within, that quiet space we all long for. Once you've tasted the sweet nectar of that stillness, once you've connected with it, you'll be hooked. And while we're not to be attached to the "fruits" of our practice, the experience of stillness keeps us coming back for more. This is where your practice can become a dangerous addiction, used as an escape from life. If we look at our time on the mat as a time-out, a time to heal, a time to reflect and do the self-study needed to change bad habits—and most importantly, change unhealthy thinking patterns—then we will get the full benefit from our practice. Let's face it: we go through life for the most part at full speed, not really taking the time to smell the roses.

Stop.

Breathe.

Enjoy life.

That's what Yoga teaches us. The practice is not meant to be an escape from life.

We do not live to do Yoga; we do Yoga to live.

> "In the beginning God created the heaven and the earth. And the earth was without form, and void; and darkness was upon the face of the deep"
> (Genesis 1:1–2, KJV).

But remember, the only things that separate us from one another are degrees of light and dark.

> "I am the Way, the Truth, and the Life"
> (John 14:6 King James Version).

When I started on my Yoga journey, it was out of necessity for my own sanity. I was in a very dark place, mentally and physically. My life was falling apart from the inside out. I had withdrawn from life. I spent a great deal of time on my own, in my own mind. I blamed my past, my parents, and my upbringing for the misery I was experiencing. To be clear, at the time the blame was not on a conscious level. I spent countless hours going over all the wrongs I thought had been done to me, and that pattern of thinking added to the misery I was feeling. As the famous Descartes quote goes, "I think, therefore I am." This quote has also been interpreted as "I think, therefore I exist." In my case, I thought I was a victim, *so I was* a victim, and I acted accordingly. The suffering was very real: I had panic attacks, nightmares, social anxiety, and feelings of distrust toward others and myself. I didn't trust my own instincts, my own feelings, or my own insight. On a physical level, I was exhausted. In a nutshell, I was *pathetic!* There were days when I had to force myself out of bed in the morning to go to work and function on a daily basis. I was the perfect victim. On the outside, I appeared to be strong, put together, and well-adjusted. I had learned at an early age how to survive, how to adjust, and how to push my feelings deep inside. I had learned to cope with stress, how to put on a smiley face, while inside I was seething with disgust for myself, frustrated by pain and a feeling of hopelessness I couldn't shake. It was getting increasingly difficult to put on the smiley face, and the frustrations of my lifetime were about to surface.

Life has a way of pushing those feelings out little by little, like putting a kettle on slow boil. Eventually it will come to a full rolling boil and those unresolved conflicts and feelings will surface. Please don't misunderstand; I'm not diminishing the effects that my childhood or the choices I was making had on my current condition, nor am I suggesting that real suffering isn't a direct result of being abused and mistreated, because it is. What I am saying is that once those effects became conscious, I had the power to shift my thinking, and with that shift, make different choices than the preconditioned ones I had been making. My practice gave me the courage to do whatever I felt necessary to heal, and it gave me the knowledge to look at my past in a different light. Changing those patterns wasn't easy, and there are days when I still struggle with old ghosts from the past. But I no longer see myself as a victim, and I know I can choose differently, even if that choice is simply how I view a situation. In doing so, I shift the energy in myself, and that in turn changes the way I deal with others and the way they deal with me in any given situation.

The practice of Yoga teaches us to take responsibility for our life and the current condition it is in. Many things can teach us these lessons, so what makes Yoga unique? How do the poses and the breathing lead to this outcome? During my training, I talked a lot about the benefits of Yoga to my family. My dad said to me one day, "You would have gotten the same benefits from anything you put that much energy into." I thought about that for a few seconds and quickly retorted with, "No, Dad, this is different." During my very first Yoga class, I shared my experience with the group. "Oh my God," I said. "I can be still, I can just rest, I'm not anyone's mother or daughter or wife right now. I'm just me, and I'm going to lay here and just be still. In the practices of Yoga, I found God! And in doing so, I realized that I am not separate from him/her/it but part of the whole of all of creation. This knowledge brings with it a comfort like no other I have ever experienced. In the silence of meditation, I realized that I was causing my own suffering as well as causing those around me to suffer.

I am certain that many have found this in similar spiritual practices, but I personally found this in Yoga! I had tried other practices, although I used these as a form of escape from what I was feeling: art courses, different churches, exercise programs, work, trying to be the perfect daughter or have the perfect bod. These were all attempts to escape feeling. Let me ask you this: When did you last feel calm, at peace, and content? Ironically, once I was quiet long enough to hear that voice within, I became much more content with all the roles of mother, daughter, and wife because I realized they are not who I truly am. I no longer felt the need to run away from myself; instead, I felt the need to turn my attention inward, back toward the self. This is what separates Yoga from other practices, beyond the obvious physical benefits. To find this, you must be still and go within to the space of silence we call the Gap.

Everything is a choice. I can choose to react in a negative manner to any given situation, or I can step back and look at the situation from a different vantage point. That allows me to make a conscious choice, though it's not always easy to make conscious choices. Sometimes a situation pulls us in so quickly that we find ourselves responding in a negative manner, falling back into old patterns of behaviour. When that happens, it's easy to find judgement in our behaviour, but this serves no purpose. Patience and perseverance will prevail in our practice. Those old patterns of acting and reacting can be replaced by new productive ones. Reprograming our old patterns takes time and effort, but it's well worth it. Each new seed of choice nurtures new patterns that will yield positive results, creating a new Karmic pattern.

Learning to stay present takes practice. Far too often, we don't live in the present moment; our minds wander to the past or the future. Rarely do we stay present in the moment. Staying present allows us to live, *truly live*, not just exist. The famous country music singer Keith Urban did a tour a few years back called "Be Here." I remember thinking, *Be where?* Now I get it. Be present ... just be! The Gap allows us to do this. How much we miss by being stuck in our own heads, in our own judgements and prejudices. Bring to mind the most beautiful flower you can think of. The flower is what it is; it grows from a seed into a full-grown flower, and the flower doesn't care if the next flower beside it is bigger or smaller, or whether or not the adjacent flower has more colour or less. It doesn't even care if the flower beside it gets more sunlight or gets picked first. It exists for what it is—no more, no less.

We as humans should do the same.

Let's return to our main question in this chapter: What is Yoga? It's extremely hard to narrow down. If you think of Yoga as a gigantic tree that has been growing for thousands of years with roots that run deep with the knowledge passed down from the gods, you have just touched the surface. For as many individuals as there are in this world, there are branches in that tree, and what works for one person may not work for another. The beauty is that you can just go to another branch and keep going until you find the one that works for you.

If "Yoga" means to unite, or to *yuk*, and bring mind, body, and breath in alignment with our true nature, then we must ask: What is our true nature? We have gotten so far away from nature: living and working in our concrete boxes, eating processed foods, and demanding instant gratification! Yoga is a means to come back ... back to nature, in a sense. On a much deeper level, our true nature, according to the Yoga philosophy, is not our bodies, our gender, our social status, or our religious beliefs but the eternal part of our being that is born into this body and will leave this body upon our last breath. The practice of Yoga is said to reveal this truth, this *Vidya,* or knowledge of the true self.

According to the father of Yoga, Patañjali, who is said to have codified Yoga, Yoga is the stilling of the fluctuations of the mind. In other words, shutting up the monkey in our brains, the thought waves that control our behaviour. Our behaviour becomes our character, and our character becomes our destiny. We are the thought waves of our mind, and if our thoughts are harmful, we suffer. "In the beginning was the Word" (John 1:1). The concept here is that God had a thought to create light from darkness, and the thought precedes the action. Perhaps if God had not had the thought first, all would still be darkness. Before life, or manifested life, was consciousness, and from consciousness came the Word. It has been my experience that people identify closely with the mind as being the master of our lives, without awareness of their true selves. Have you ever tried to shut up your thoughts? Not so easy, is it? But with practice and the discipline of Yoga, you can learn to master your thoughts. Remember, Yoga as I understand it is the uniting of the mind, body, and breath, connecting with the Divine. Nothing is separate from the whole—not you, not me, not anything in existence. Within each of us exists everything. In a sense, we *are* the universe.

I have never found more peace in this life than what I've found in surrendering to the practice on my mat. Surrender is an important part of the practice, and one that I feel many will resist. We're more likely as humans to keep trying to control everything around us so that we feel safe. My previous search for God—as I understood him or her at the time—was in vain.

I searched in chapels, in spiritual texts, in pastors, etc. I followed the doctrine and prayed, but there was something missing. My soul wasn't satisfied, and the million questions I had in my head were never answered, until I started looking within. If you're waiting for someone, some God outside yourself, to make you happy, you'll be waiting an exceptionally long time. But when you sit still and take a deep breath, you may find yourself suddenly in awe: you have found God! The peace that surpasses all understanding exists inside of you! Lay down your sword and let the pain of your heart go! Breathe and know that *you* are God, and you are good enough! You are Yoga! How often do you feel unworthy, unloved, or just not good enough, especially in the presence of God? Yoga allows you to create the space within your consciousness to reconnect to your higher self, to your true nature, which is infinitely more than the role you play in this life— not your gender, your age, or your social status, but that part of you that existed before you were born and that part of you that will carry on when this body is worn out.

In making the decision to begin your Yoga journey, an important step is finding the Yoga that's right for you. The main types of Yoga are *Karma Yoga* (which we discussed earlier) *Bhakti Yoga, Jnana Yoga,* and *Raja Yoga.* We'll explore each in turn. There are a number of other types of Yoga here in North America that are very different than the traditional Yogas we're about to explore. You may be more familiar with Hot Yoga, Hatha Yoga, or Iyengar Yoga.

The Main Types of Yoga

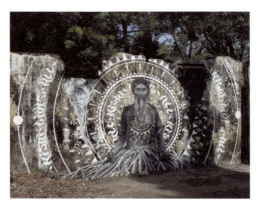

Bhakti Yoga

Bhakti Yoga is the Yoga of devotion: "Those who fix their minds on Me and always engage in My devotion with steadfast faith, I consider them to be the best yogis" (*Bhagavad Gita* 12:2). With the practice of Bhakti Yoga, the individual should not have any expectations of any rewards. This follows closely with the practice of Karma Yoga and not being attached to the outcome. Bhakti Yoga is widely practised by the Indian masses. I believe that most individuals in the West start Yoga as an exercise program, or with the intention of finding peace of mind from relaxation techniques that reduce stress. Through practice, even with little effort, they eventually realize that we are not our bodies. Once they discover that there is more to our existence than meets the eye, it only makes sense that the natural progression would be a cultivation of reverence for the divine inside and outside of ourselves.

---

17 Image by Audrey O'Marra, "All you need is love....", as posted to *Facebook,* 23 January 2019. https://www.facebook.com/photo.php?fbid=10215608015727683&set= pb.1059544614.-2207520000..&type=3

One way to practise Bhakti Yoga is to visualize God or the Divine sitting or standing before you and then focus with intensity on your feelings of love and devotion to God. God has wired us to reach out to him, and the heart is the pathway to the divine. Below are some important quotes applicable to Bhakti Yoga:

"The heart is intimately connected with every facet of the body and brain through its own neural extensions."[18]

"Trust what is not known to your Mind. Trust what is known to your Heart."[19]

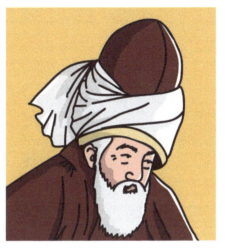

[20]

"Don't grieve. Anything you lose comes round in another form …
Let the beauty of what you love be what you do …
Only from the heart can you touch the sky."[21]

---

[18] J.C. Pearce, *The Biology of Transcendence: A Blueprint of the Human Spirit* (New York, NY: Simon and Shuster, 2004). shorturl.at/dhovQ

[19] This quote is attributed to Tony Samara. https://tonysamara.com/about/.

[20] Jalāl ad-Dīn Muhammad Rūmī (known more popularly simply as Rumi), a thirteenth-century Persian poet, Hanafi faqih, Islamic scholar, Maturidi theologian, and Sufi mystic.

[21] Coleman Barks (trans.), *The Essential Rumi* (NJ: Castle Books, 1997), 272.

Jnana Yoga

Jnana Yoga is the Yoga of wisdom and spiritual knowledge. The individual uses their intellect and knowledge to come to the awareness of the Divine. Through the practice of meditation and not allowing the distractions of emotions or thoughts to interfere, one breaks the veil of ignorance. The practice of *neti-neti*, which means "neither this nor that,"[22] while meditating or going about your daily routine helps to overcome restless thoughts. It means not becoming attached to the thoughts or feelings when they arise, just as we shouldn't be attached to rewards in Karma Yoga. One practice that has worked for me when I catch my mind in a loop of thoughts is saying, "Thinking, you are thinking again." This is a helpful tool to negate negative mind chatter.

In using the mind as a tool for practising Jnana Yoga, one shouldn't confuse the mind with the ego. The mind may *witness* a thought, but the ego *attaches* itself to it. I may have a thought that may induce an emotion of some kind. If I take that thought and run with it, it leads to another thought, which leads to more emotions and responses in the physical body. If I use my mind to discern if that thought is useful or not, I don't give my ego the chance to respond. Neither this, nor that! This is the practice of self-study; we study our thoughts to determine which thoughts are useful and which are not. When a thought provokes a strong emotional response, we learn not to get caught up in that emotion but to let the energy it creates run its course without fuelling it anymore. We also must not resist the emotions; we don't want to stuff them down again but rather allow them the space to clear.

Swami Vivekananda says, "To get any reason out of the mass of incongruity we call human life, we have to transcend our reason, but we must do it

---

[22] S. O'Donnell, "What is Neti-Neti?" *Hridaya Yoga Blog,* November 13, 2017, https://hridaya-Yoga.com/what-is-neti-neti/.

scientifically, slowly, by regular practice, and we must cast off all superstition."[23] This is the practice of Jnana Yoga, the Yoga of Wisdom! Swami Vivekananda was an Indian Hindu monk who was a key figure in the introduction of the Indian philosophies of Yoga to the Western world. He is credited with raising interfaith awareness and bringing Hinduism to the status of a major world religion in the nineteenth century.[24] He's perhaps best known for his speech in which he introduced Hinduism at the Parliament of the World's Religions in Chicago in 1893.

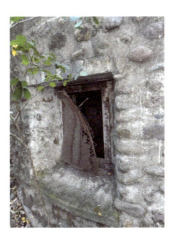

"Sisters and Brothers of America,
It fills my heart with joy unspeakable to rise in response to the warm and cordial welcome which you have given us. I thank you in the name of the most ancient order of monks in the world; I thank you in the name of the mother of religions, and I thank you in the name of millions and millions of Hindu people of all classes and sects."[25]

---

[23] S. Vivekananda, *The Complete Works of Swami Vivekananda, Volume I: Addresses at the Parliament of Religions, Karma-Yoga, Raja-Yoga, Lectures and Discourses* (New York: Discovery, 2017),

[24] P.B. Clarke, *New Religions in Global Perspective*. (Oxfordshire, UK: Routledge, 2006), 209.

[25] H. Dutt, *Immortal Speeches: New Delhi*. (London, UK: Unicorn Books, 2005), 121.

Raja Yoga

Raja Yoga is considered royal because the Yogi who practises this Yoga thereby becomes ruler of his mind.[26] Raja Yoga is the Yoga of Meditation: using meditation to reach higher consciousness. While some paths of Yoga advocate bringing the body under control by postures, proper diet, and moral restraints to purify the system enough to be able to reach *Samadhi*, the practice of Raja Yoga approaches it from the opposite viewpoint: by bringing the mind under control with the practice of meditation, we bring the body under control. In order to do that, we must follow the eight-limb process as set out by Patañjali. But if the body isn't healthy, how can we sit in meditation? This seems a bit contradictory, to say the least.

According to the teachings of Patañjali, if we follow the eight limbs of Yoga, we will attain higher consciousness. This higher consciousness is the goal of all serious Yogis; it is not about holding an asana or having the perfect Yoga body. We will explore Raja Yoga through the Patañjali Sūtras.

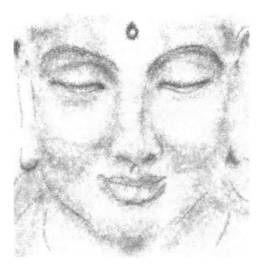

---

[26] Yoga Association of Seychelles, *Branches of Yoga.*
http://Yogaassociationofseychelles.weebly.com/about-Yoga.html

The compiler of the *Yoga Sūtras* and a notable scholar of Hindu philosophy,[27] Patañjali is estimated to have lived between the second and fourth century CE.[28] His work is considered the foundation of Yoga[29] and one of the most important texts in Indian culture, having been translated into no less than forty different languages.[30]

According to Patañjali, the definition of Yoga is, *Yogas citta vritti nirodhah*, meaning "Yoga is the restraint of fluctuations/patterns of consciousness."[31] In simpler terms, "Yoga is the control of the thought waves in the mind."[32] The thought waves of the mind constantly fluctuate, and Yoga practice is "the steadfast effort to still these fluctuations."[33] The goal of Yoga, then, is to find our true self, "to unlearn the false identification of the thought waves with the ego-sense."[34] But what is our true self? If we aren't our bodies or the roles we play in this life, what are we? When we get caught up in thought waves, we're not living in the present moment; we are either worrying about the future or

---

[27] S. H. Phillips, *Yoga, Karma, and Rebirth: A Brief History and Philosophy* (New York, NY: Columbia University Press, 2013).

[28] E.F. Bryant, *The Yoga Sūtras of Patañjali: A New Edition, Translation and Commentary* (New York: North Point Press, 2009).

[29] M.M. Desmarais, *Changing Minds: Mind, Consciousness, and Identity in Patañjali's Yoga-Sūtra and Cognitive Neuroscience* (New Delhi: Motilal Banarsidass, 2008), 15–16.

[30] D.G. White, *The Yoga Sūtra of Patañjali: A Biography.* (Princeton, NJ: Princeton University Press, 2014).

[31] S. Radhakrishnan and C.A. Moore, *A Source Book in Indian Philosophy* (Princeton, NJ: Princeton University Press, 1989).

[32] M. Jacuzzi, "Patañjali's Conception of the Mind," *Seven Winds Yoga & Jyotish,* 2005, http://www.sevenwindsYoga.com/writing/articles/Patañjali-s-conception-of-the-mind

[33] B.K.S. Iyengar, *Light on the Yoga Sūtras of Patañjali* (New York, NY: HarperCollins, 1993), 61.

[34] S. Prabhavananda, « Patañjali Yoga Sūtras, » *Sri Ramakrishna Math,* 1953, 4, https://estudantedavedanta.net/Yoga-Aphorisms-of-Patanjali.pdf

fretting over the past. In order to achieve the goal of finding our true self, we need a clear understanding of the foundation of Yoga. The Patañjali Sūtras are that foundation.

I wouldn't expect anyone to take a road trip to an unknown place without a guide or map. Patañjali has mapped the path for those individuals who want to achieve higher consciousness and find their true nature. He has laid out the foundation of not only the obstacles that prevent us from finding our true nature—which is God—but he has also given us alternative practices to replace old habits with new ones, and a method to overcome those obstacles, which can include depression, sadness, irregular breathing habits, and so on.

With the practice of meditation and the surrender to *Īśvara* ("The Lord," another name for the Supreme Soul or God),[35] we can find union with our true self.

Even if your goal isn't to find union with "God," per se, at the very least you have a framework to go by to still your restless mind and live a life in the present moment, where all the magic exists. You can read the texts, travel to distant lands, and search out teachers, but *you* and *only you* must do the work of self-discovery and self-analysis.

Patañjali writes that "*Īśvarapraṇidhāna,* devotional surrender to God" is "a prerequisite to meditational Yoga" and that "*Īśvara* is represented by the mystical syllable 'om'... It is through the sound *om* that the yogi is to fix the mind on *Īś*vara:

"By constantly repeating *om* and contemplating its meaning, *artha*, namely *Īśvara* [God], the mind of the *yogi* becomes one-pointed – the goal of all *Yoga* practice. Repeating the sound *om* and "contemplating its meaning," namely, that it is the sound representation of *Īśvara* [God], the object of the *yogi's* surrender, when coupled with Patañjali's usage of the word *praṇidhāna,* surrender, in I.23, points to chanting the mantra in a devotional mood. This is

---

[35] H.P. Sullivan, s.v. "Isvara," *Encyclopedia of Religion* (New York: MacMillan Publishing, 1987), 498–499.

quintessential Hindu theistic meditation, the most prominent form of Hindu Yoga evidenced from antiquity to the present day".[36]

Chanting *om,* the sound of God, leads to surrendering ourselves to *Isvara,* free from *vritti* (thought waves) and karmas. In other words, meditation on God with the repetition of *om* removes obstacles to the mastery of the inner self.

I should perhaps reiterate here a key point among all this talk of connection to and sounds of God: Yoga itself is not a religion, despite being deeply rooted in the Hindu practices of India. These are the Hindu theistic elements of Yoga, to borrow the phrasing above. In your Yoga practice, you can focus on any being of your choice—Jesus, Patañjali, the Buddha, etc. The focus of the Yoga journey is to the divine *within,* to the source of all creation. Some people use the term universe, I use the term God, as does Patañjali through the name *Īśvara.* Regardless of the name you use, the emphasis in Yoga is on stilling the thoughts in our minds. But in order to still them, we must understand them and their roots.

According to the teachings of Patañjali, there are five different types of thought waves. I bet you thought you only had to worry about one! Don't be discouraged; we'll explore each of them in depth. Some of these are considered painful, while others are not.

---

[36] E. Bryant, "The Yoga Sūtras of Patañjali," *Internet Encyclopedia of Philosophy,* https://iep.utm.edu/Yoga/.

The Five Types of Thought Waves (or Modifications of the Mind)[37]

1. *Pramana*, meaning "right [correct] knowledge"
2. *Viparyaya*, meaning "wrong [incorrect] knowledge"
3. *Vikalpa*, meaning "imagination"
4. *Nidra*, meaning "sleep" or "emptiness"
5. *Smrtaya*, meaning "memory"

Pramana, Right Knowledge

This thought wave is considered "right knowledge," according to Patañjali. These are the thoughts that direct the mind toward greater knowledge and freedom from suffering. The right knowledge thoughts (*Pramana*) are direct perception, inference, and scriptural or revealed authority. With the right thought process, you can determine right knowledge based on sensory input. An example of direct perception would be placing your hand on a hot burner and feeling the pain of the burn. The mind reacts and pulls the hand away. Even with right knowledge, there can be pain. Metaphorically, we continue to do things that bring us pain even with the right perception. This is where the deeper self-analysis is needed in order to change old habits and prevent ourselves from metaphorically placing our hand on the hot burner time and time again.

Viparyaya, Wrong Knowledge

Those thought waves that carry a false perception of an object and don't correspond with its real form are considered "wrong knowledge." You may see an

---

[37] G.B. Abbott, "The 5 Kinds of Modifications of the Mind," *Original Christianity and Original Yoga*, April 27, 2014, https://ocoy.org/the-5-kinds-of-modifications-of-the-mind/

object and perceive it to be something other than what it is, and that perception may cause a negative response. An example of this would be the classic "rope being perceived as a snake," causing a reaction of fear and a response to flee from the object or attack it. The "monsters under the bed" can be a combination of *Viparyaya* and *Vikalpa*, or imagination. They are always the monsters in our head! When we feel that type of reaction, we fight, fly, or freeze. If this perception becomes a normal response to the world around us, our bodies eventually wear down.

Vikalpa, Imagination

According to Patañjali, imagination is the thoughts that are made up in the mind without an external object, or when the verbal does not match with reality. I think a large majority of individuals struggle with this every day—drawing a conclusion based on what they thought they heard, when the person saying the words meant something entirely different. Imagination isn't always a bad thing; it's the source of creation as well. All artists and scientists use some sort of imagination to bring an idea to life. But in the context of Yoga, we are training the mind to stay in the present moment and learn to determine the real from the unreal.

Nidra, Sleep or Emptiness

These are the thoughts, according to Patañjali, that are in the absence of cognition or the process of being aware of thought. They're usually made in the mind during sleep, or while in a dream-like state.

Smrtaya, Memory

Memory is those thoughts that are stored in the mind from experience and can be brought back to consciousness. I sometimes think of the mind as a filing cabinet in which we store the thoughts away for future use. But even these thoughts are subjective to our perceptions, and each time we remember, the experience changes a bit.[38] Talk to any two people who experienced the same event, and you'll hear completely different versions.

So where does this leave us? In my personal experience, it takes great effort and practice to not only be aware of the thought waves (*vrittis*) of the mind (*citta*) on a conscious level, but also to take the steps necessary to control them. It has also been my experience that you can't control your thoughts per se, but you *can* become a master of being aware of them. You can't change your responses to your thoughts if you're not aware of them. In my own practice, as thoughts of fear and anger or any other *viparyaya* arise, I try to catch myself and replace those thoughts with ones of compassion and understanding for the individual or situation I perceive is causing me such pain, and also for myself by not judging myself but looking at the situation in a detached way. That's easier said than done, but with practice and determination, you'll build the skills necessary to control those thoughts.

At times I recognize that I would enjoy nothing better than acting out some of my negative thoughts. I have to constantly remind myself that when I react to my thoughts in a negative manner, or when I become defensive, those reactions are not part of my true nature. They're part of my ego-self and could be caused by some triggers from my past, or past lives, that need to be brought to my awareness. At times what appears to be *pramana* is in fact *viparyaya*. The desire for a new home, a new job, or a new mate may seem at the time not to cause pain, but they may have painful consequences down the road. Perhaps upon acquiring the new house, job, or mate, I realize that the desire was short-lived, which causes me despair. That burger that looks so good and gives me

---

[38] A. Dobrin, "Your Memory Isn't What You Think It Is," *Psychology Today,* July 16, 2013, https://www.psychologytoday.com/ca/blog/am-i-right/201307/your-memory-isnt-what-you-think-it-is.

pleasure while eating it also gives me a stomach-ache and clogged arteries down the road. On the other hand, what at first appears to be painful, like ending an unhealthy relationship, may bring you peace and harmony down the road. To become conscious of your choices, you must trust and have faith that with practice and detachment, you will overcome the fluctuations of your mind.

Patañjali offers several ways to eliminate or control the *vrittis* of the *citta*, such as total surrender to the Divine with the practice of *om* (also called the *Pranava Mantra*). If this is practised with devotion and total surrender, the mind will be freed from its fluctuations. As Patañjali states, "At that time (the time of concentration) the seer (Purusha) rests in his own (unmodified) state. At other times (other than that of concentration) the seer is identified with the modifications".[39] Meditation on God, or any object, with single-minded effort will still the mind. By regulating our breathing, we have the means to control the thoughts in our minds.[40]

According to Patañjali (Sūtra 2.29), The Eight Limbs of Yoga are:

1. *Yamas*—Moral Principles
2. *Niyamas*—Observances
3. *Sana*—Postures
4. *Prānāyāma*—Control of the Breath
5. *Pratyāhāra*—Going Within
6. *Dhāranā* – Concentration
7. *Dhyāna*—Meditation
8. *Samādhi*—Absorption

---

[39] Swami Vivekananda's translations of Sūtra 1.3 and 1.4, according to Yoga Sūtra Study (2021). YSP-Sūtras 1.01-1.20. Chapter 1: "Samadhi Pada," *Yoga Sūtra Study: Path to Enlightenment,* https://yogasutrastudy.info/yoga-sutra-translations/ysp-sutras1-01-1-20/

[40] M. Perrotta, "Controlling Your Mind by Controlling Your Breath," *The Startup*, June 10, 2020, https://medium.com/swlh/neuroscience-of-breath-63c32604be22.

The Eight Limbs of Yoga

1. <u>*Yamas*</u>: moral principles, the self-disciplines or self-restraints of Yoga practice. Similar to the Ten Commandments of the Bible, they include *Ahimsa* (non-violence), *Satyam* (truthfulness), *Asteya* (honesty), *Brahmacarya* (continence), and *Aparigraha* (non-possessiveness). Moral practices include abstinence from immoral behaviours.
2. <u>*Niyamas*</u>: observances, the ways one should treat themselves. They include *Sauca* (purity), *Samtosa* (contentment), *Tapas* (the inner heat of effort), *Svadhyaya* (self-analysis), and *Īśvarapraṇidhāna* (surrender to God).
3. <u>*Āsana*</u>: postures, sitting in preparation for meditation; being alert and relaxed and steady in sitting to the point that it becomes effortless.[41]
4. <u>*Prāṇāyāma*</u>: the control of our breath. By learning to control our breath, we learn to calm our minds. This also promotes awareness of the life force that is *prana,* a universal energy that flows in currents in and around the body.[42]
5. <u>*Pratyāhāra*</u>: detachment, the art of watching from a distance in the mind and not being attached to the senses. It empowers one to stop being controlled by the external world and experience the freedom innate in one's inner world.[43]

---

[41] H. Āraṇya, *Yoga Philosophy of Patañjali* (Albany, NY: State University of New York Press, 1983), 229.

[42] M. Ramamurti, *Fundamentals of Yoga*, 2nd Ed. (New York: Baba Bhagavandas Publication Trust, 2002), 216.

[43] R.S. Bajpai, *The Splendours and Dimensions of Yoga.* (New Delhi: Motilal Banarsidass, 2002), 342-345.

6. *Dhāranā*: concentration, consciously focusing on one object to avoid other thoughts.
7. *Dhyāna*: meditation, stilling the thoughts of the mind in order to focus on the present moment.
8. *Samādhi*: absorption of or becoming one with your object of meditation (*Atman* or God).

The desire or intention of practice is to reach Atman. In order to reach Atman, the mind must be stilled, and the Eight Limbs provide the practices necessary to still the mind

According to Patañjali, the *Yamas* and the *Niyamas* are the primary principles of morality and are the first two limbs of the Eight Limbs of Yoga. You could compare them to the Ten Commandments of the Bible in the sense that they are moral guidelines to be followed.[44] We will begin with the *Yamas,* the moral principles that constitute the first of the Eight Limbs of Yoga.

1. *Ahimsa*, meaning "non-injury" or "non-harm"
2. *Satyam*, meaning "truthfulness"
3. *Asteya*, meaning "honesty," "not stealing," "not coveting"
4. *Brahmacarya*, meaning "continence"
5. *Aparigraha*, meaning "non-possessiveness," "non-attachment"

Ahimsa means to bring no harm and to abstain from violence, which includes not only acts of violence but violent thoughts.[45] Some take this to the extreme, taking great measures to harm nothing, including the smallest of creatures, so they don't walk on grass for fear of breaking a blade.

---

[44] J. Lasater, "Beginning the Journey," *Yoga Journal*, Issue 6, 1998, 42–48.
[45] J.G. Lochtefeld, "Yama (2)," *The Illustrated Encyclopedia of Hinduism*, Vol. 2 (New York, NY: Rosen Publishing, 2000), 777.

Satyam means truthfulness, being honest with oneself and others, and always speaking the truth. However, "speaking the truth" excludes truths that would bring harm to others.[46]

Asteya means non-stealing, including coveting something that is not yours. Asteya isn't merely "theft by action." It also includes "theft by intent" and/or "manipulation." Persistent exploitation of the weak or poor is a form of "Asteya in one's thought."[47]

Brahmacarya: "The fourth vow—brahmacarya—means for laypersons, marital fidelity and pre-marital celibacy; for ascetics, it means absolute celibacy.[48] John Cort explains, 'Brahmacharya [for the average person] involves having sex only with one's spouse, as well as the avoidance of ardent gazing or lewd gestures.'"[49]

Aparigraha means "non-possessiveness," or "non-attachment." We should only possess what we need, and not hoard. Our possessions don't define our happiness or our true nature. This is similar to *Asteya,* but Asteya refers to the possessions of others, while *Aparigraha* refers to one's own property, including not accepting improper gifts offered by others, non-avarice, and non-craving in the motivation of one's deeds, words, and thoughts.[50]

Next are the *Niyamas,* the observances that constitute the second of the Eight Limbs of Yoga.

---

[46] A. Dhand, "The dharma of ethics, the ethics of dharma: Quizzing the ideals of Hinduism," *Journal of Religious Ethics*, 2002, 30(3), 347-372.

[47] N.A. Nikam, "Gandhi's Philosophy," *The Review of Metaphysics*, 1954, Vol. 7(4), 668-678.

[48] J. Long, *Jainism: An Introduction.* (London, UK: IB Tauris, 2009), 109.

[49] Quoted in Long (2009), 101. Brackets added by me.

[50] J. Wood, *The Yoga System of Patañjali* (Cambridge, MA: Harvard University Press, 1914), 178-182.

The Niyamas

1. *Sauca*, meaning "purity"
2. *Samtosa*, meaning "contentment"
3. *Tapas*, literally "inner heat," meaning "effort"
4. *Svadhyaya*, meaning "self-study"
5. *Īśvarapraṇidhāna*, meaning "surrender to God"

Sauca literally means purity, cleanliness, and clearness. It refers to purity of mind, speech, and body. Anger, hate, prejudice, greed, pride, and fear are examples of impurity of mind.[51] One's body is considered a temple of God, as in the teachings of Christianity: "Do you not know that your bodies are temples of the Holy Spirit, who is in you, whom you have received from God?" (1 Corinthians 6:19, New International Version).

Samtosa means being content with what one has in the present moment and showing gratitude for one's circumstances, even if those circumstances seem unpleasant. It's the habit of accepting one's circumstances without being upset.[52]

Tapas refers to the "inner heat" caused by the effort of self-discipline. This heat purifies the system and destroys impurities in the same way that heating different metals destroys their impurities.[53]

Svadhyaya, you might recall from earlier, means self-study or self-analysis. If you don't know yourself, you can't make the necessary changes to raise your level of awareness to break through the veils of ignorance and reach the Atman, or God.

---

[51] K.V. Raghupathi, K.V. (2007). *Yoga for Peace* (India, Abhinav Publications, 2007), 60–61.

[52] A. Daniélou, *Yoga: Mastering the Secrets of Matter and the Universe*. (Rochester, VT: Inner Traditions, 1991), 36.

[53] G. Bailey and I. Mabbett, *The Sociology of Early Buddhism* (Cambridge, UK: Cambridge University Press, 2003), 152.

Finally, *Īśvarapraṇidhāna* (represented by *om*), means to surrender to God by living in dedication to God and turning your life over to the divine. That divine is different for each of us.

Applying the Yamas and Niyamas to Everyday Life

As I contemplated the *Yamas* and *Niyamas* and how I could apply them in my own practice, I realized that I have a lot of work ahead of me.

At first glance, my ego-self thought, *I don't bring harm to anyone, and I'm an honest person. If someone gives me too much change, I give it back. I balance my cheque book. I pay my bills on time. I don't covet—well, at least I try to make a conscious effort not to—and when it comes to continence, well, I am in my fifties. Sex just isn't on the top of my priority list*. With all this in mind, I thought I was good to go. But there lies the problem: we are what our thoughts are.

While I don't intentionally harm, and I certainly don't go out of my way to hurt others, I do catch myself having what could be considered harmful thoughts. There are certain people in my life that repulse me, and their actions trigger a response in me that isn't what I would consider godly. When I hear a co-worker gossiping about others, or enjoying the pain they cause others, my first reaction is one of anger and frustration. Instead, I should be seeing past their level of awareness to their true nature. While I don't steal, there are times that I steal time, like checking my email at work. While sex isn't at the top of my priority list, I'm well aware of the side of me that is very sensual and enjoys the pleasure sex brings, while knowing that giving that energy away is like giving away a piece of my soul.

While I'm not possessive in the sense that I believe that my possessions dictate my happiness, I have attachments to my routine, my schedule, my lists. I like order and knowing what I'm doing. In starting this journey, I have changed my morning routine; I didn't realize just how attached I was to it until then. Reflecting on how I can apply the *Yamas* to my practice, I must be patient and non-judgemental in order to gain control over my ego and continue to practise them on a conscious level.

When these negative thoughts and feelings surface, they must be replaced with ones of love and compassion. While practising my meditation, I must begin with the intentions of a pure heart, continually making the effort to set aside time for practice and study of the scriptures, as well as for self-study. By bringing these practices and observances to the mat every day, they will overflow to my life.

In the end, the surrender to the Divine—having faith that, ultimately, God will guide my path in this life—is the connection with the Divine that I seek. It was surrender that brought me to this Eight-Limbed path!

The Eight Limbs of Yoga are the central tenets of the practice, but there are a few more important terms and types of Yoga that students and teachers should be mindful of.

Term: Kleshas[54]

The *Kleshas* are the five afflictions or obstacles of the mind that prevent us from being able to *yuk* (unite) with God. These include *Avidya* (ignorance), *Asmita* (the ego), *Raga* (attachments), *Dvesa* (aversions), and *Abhinivesa* (fear of death).

1. *Avidya*, meaning "ignorance," is a lack of spiritual knowledge; the misunderstanding that we perceive ourselves as separate from the source of our true identity, which is oneness with God. We came from wholeness, and we return to wholeness.

---

[54] L.D. Angerame, L.D. (2017). "The Kleshas: Five Obstacles to Awareness," *Embodied Philosophy*, Issue 1, April 9, 2017, https://www.embodiedphilosophy.com/the-kleshas-five-obstacles-to-awareness-2/

2. *Asmita*, meaning "ego," refers to identifying who we are with our ego, the "I" self, and believing that our ego represents our true selves.
3. *Raga*, meaning "attachment," refers to our attachment to what we believe may bring us happiness and security; we grasp for higher social status, more money, and more belongings, perceiving these will bring us peace of mind.
4. *Dvesa*, meaning "aversion," refers to when the external pleasures we desire don't bring us the lasting happiness or contentment we think they should. We then begin to dislike or hate them, causing ourselves pain.
5. *Abhinivesa*, meaning "fear of death," refers to our attachment to being alive, usually fuelled by uncertainty of what will become of our spirits when our bodies expire on Earth.

More Types of Yoga

We have devoted most of this chapter to the principles of Raja Yoga, but other types of Yoga are also mentioned in the Patañjali Sūtras.

Kriya Yoga is a combination of the practice of Raja Yoga, Jnana Yoga, and Bhakti Yoga. "Austerity, the study of sacred texts, and the dedication of action to God constitute the discipline of Mystic Union."[55] The Patañjali Sūtra refers to the practice of Kriya Yoga as a "burning zeal in practice, self-study and study of scriptures, and surrender to God."[56] Kriya Yoga is considered an ancient prac-

---

[55] K. Keegan, "Sutra 2.1: The Basics of Spiritual Discipline and Intro to Book 2" *No Big Secret Yoga & Astrology,* April 30, 2015. http://no-bsyoga.com/keeganlife/2015/04/sutra-21.html

[56] N. Barnes, "What is the significance of Patanjali's Sūtra 2.1?" *Blogger,* September 3, 2011, http://nielanbarnesYoga.blogspot.com/2011/09/what-is-significance-of-patanjalis.html

tice, as many of its references come from the texts of the Bhagavad-Gita and the Patañjali Sūtras.

According to Patañjali, the purpose of Kriya Yoga is to reduce the effects of afflictions (*Kleshas*) on the mind, therefore making it easier to reach *Samadhi*. Kriya Yoga focuses on three of the *Niyamas*. First is *Tapas* (inner heat, effort), which in this context applies to the physical practice, self-discipline, eating habits, moral discipline, and postures associated with Kriya Yoga. This is the "burning zeal in practice" that the Patañjali Sūtras refer to: literally the inner heat of effort. The second is *Svadhyaya*, which means looking inward in order to self-study or self-analyze. This is the self-study that the Patañjali Sūtras refer to. Finally there is *Īśvarapraṇidhāna*, or "the surrender to God."

As long as we believe that external events and the acquisition of material things will bring us contentment, we will never reach Samadhi and we will continue to suffer. Recently, my daughters and I went to a country music concert to see someone I have idealized for over twenty years. Because I've listened to this artist since I was in my early twenties, my children have as well. His music has been as much a part of our lives as breathing. The experience was fantastic; we laughed and enjoyed every minute of it. While travelling home, I had never felt so tired. I had depleted my energy; I didn't do my Yoga practice, or meditation over the course of the weekend, and by Sunday evening, my brain was mush.

While I enjoyed self-gratification, my practice and self-discipline were put on the back burner, and my body let me know it. According to Patañjali, in order to break spiritual complacency, one must have trust, confidence, a sharp memory, and the power of absorption. As long as the ego is in charge, these are all exceedingly difficult to achieve. By practicing the principles of Kriya Yoga, I will conquer the ego. In my own personal practice, following the structure of Kriya Yoga will help me find the self-discipline needed to break the old habits and rid the mind of the afflictions. Because I'm aware that my ego doesn't take very long to take over, the practice of Kriya Yoga is invaluable.

<u>Tantra Yoga</u> is the practice of transforming our desires, especially our sexual desires, into energy that can be used to reach higher consciousness. While the

practice of many of the other types of Yoga focus on detaching ourselves from our desire, Tantra Yoga emphasizes those desires in an effort to transform them.

When I think of Tantra Yoga, the first thing that comes to mind are sex shops that contain books on poses I'm sure even the most practiced Yogis can't do. The union of the male and female energy has ritualistic roles in the practice of Tantric Yoga. Our Western minds are unfamiliar with a ritual that would use sexual energies to reach enlightenment. Everything in the universe is based on opposites: up/down, in/out, hot/cold, day/night, love/hate. Bringing the male/female energies into balance is one of the focuses of Tantra Yoga.

Our desires are part of our nature, and our existence depends on those desires. Without the desire to be with another, we wouldn't reproduce, and our species would soon perish! Opening these energies should be done by an individual who has already purified his mind and heart. Before attempting to practice Tantra Yoga, it's advisable to practice the Eight Limbs of Yoga for however long it takes to prepare one for such a journey!

<u>Mantra Yoga</u> is the Yoga of sound, the use of chanting, and mantras. "In the beginning was the Word" (John 1:1a). Everything in the universe is made up of vibrations. The yogi uses chanting, with the intention of clearing the mind and emotions, to reach Samadhi. This path is best suited for individuals who find it difficult to quiet the restless thoughts in their minds.

The Patañjali Sūtra states that by "constantly repeating *om* and contemplating its meaning … the mind of the yogi becomes one-pointed, which is the goal of all Yoga practice."[57] Each mantra carries with it a different energy that can be felt in the body. I often think of mantras as tuning our bodies to the energy of the divine, similar to that of a tuning fork and a musical instrument. As in all paths of Yoga, whatever mantra is chosen, the intent and attention given is most important. One mantra that I found very helpful in my practice is *Om*

---

[57] E. Bryant, "The Yoga Sūtras of Patañjali," *Internet Encyclopedia of Philosophy*, https://iep.utm.edu/Yoga/.

Gam Ganapataye Namaha,[58] or "*Om,* my salutations to Lord Ganesha."[59] This mantra is very helpful in removing obstacles from our lives.

The practice of mantras should not be taken lightly; I believe the Yoga practitioner should be very careful not to awaken such energies in the body too quickly. One should honour those who have walked the path before us and heed the teachings that have been passed down through the ages. Our modern world has instant access to ancient practices that are very powerful and, if put in the wrong hands, can be very harmful to the individual. Like the old adage says, "With great power comes great responsibility."[60] The discovery of the atom bomb is an example of great power put in the wrong hands. On the other hand, one could argue that by practising Yoga, morality happens naturally.

Hatha Yoga is my personal favourite to practise. It embodies the elements of mind, body, breath, and spirit. The practice of Hatha Yoga focuses on the purification of the body through certain disciplines, which include *asanas, pranayama*, cleaning of the body, and meditation.

From the perspective of Hatha Yoga, purification of the mind isn't possible without the purification of the body. Practising the Eight Limbs of Yoga is essential to this type of Yoga, and focus on breath is one of the key elements. The word "Hatha" comes from two roots: *ha,* which means "sun," and *tha,* which means "moon." The practice of breath control brings these hot and cold energies in the body into balance. The left nostril is said to be cool and represent the negative

---

[58] Edo & Jo—Topic, "Om Gam Ganapataye Namaha," YouTube video, 9:28, October 28, 2016, https://www.youtube.com/watch?v=F6BcPj42bUg.

[59] "Om Gam Ganapataye Namaha," *Yogapedia*, May 26, 2020, https://www.Yogapedia.com/definition/9023/om-gam-ganapataye-namaha.

[60] G. O'Toole, "With Great Power Comes Great Responsibility," *Quote Investigator,* July 23, 2015, updated July 24, 2015, https://quoteinvestigator.com/2015/07/23/great-power/.

energies in the body, while the right nostril is said to be hot, and it represents the positive energies in the body.[61]

Meditation is gaining popularity for its calming effect on the mind and body. This awareness is opening the doors for the practice of Hatha Yoga in the West. Typically, Western individuals practise this more physical type of Yoga, where the body is the focus: "The mindset in Western fitness and even Yoga has been to stretch parts like the hamstrings, and strengthen pieces with the idea that the whole body will then come together in one big, organized picture. It will not … When posture is naturally aligned, the human body stays agile without the need to do intense stretches."[62] While the body is very important in the practice of Yoga, and by strengthening and purifying the body we can set out the foundation for meditating, meditation alone will have the same affect. If you meditate on a regular basis with intent and focus, your psyche can't help but be affected.

If we were only to practise meditation, we would eventually come to know our true nature; in doing so, we would detach ourselves from the desires and negative habits that harm our bodies. We would realize that our bodies are the vehicle for the soul, and taking care of them is essential for our overall well-being.

<u>Kundalini Yoga</u> is a discipline that focuses on the awakening of the dormant energy located at the base of spine. The awakening of this energy is used to bring the individual to higher consciousness. When this Kundalini energy is awakened, it is said to travel from the base of the spine, at the *Muladhara* chakra, to the *Sahasrara* chakra, located at the crown of the head. Like the practice of Hatha Yoga, Kundalini Yoga utilizes the foundation of the Eight Limbs of Yoga to discipline the mind and body to achieve this awakening.

---

[61] R. Sovik and D. Ravizza, "Self-Study: Nostril Dominance," *Yoga International,* https://Yogainternational.com/article/view/self-study-nostril-dominance.

[62] M. Edwards, "Stop Stretching Your Hamstrings!" *Huff Post,* March 18, 2017, updated March 22, 2017, https://www.huffpost.com/entry/stop-stretching-your-hamstrings_b_58cdb802e4b0e0d348b34421

As in Kundalini Yoga, Laya Yoga focuses on the energy centres in the body known as the chakras. There are seven major energy centres located in the body:

1. The **Sahasrara** chakra is located at the crown of the head. Samādhi is achieved!
2. The **Ajna** chakra is located between the eyebrows and is the centre of connecting to life beyond the veils of ignorance (knowing our true nature beyond the body of the physical realms).
3. The **Vishuddha** chakra is located in the throat area. The element for this chakra is air. This is the centre of speaking our truths and listening to others' truths.
4. The **Anahata** chakra is located in the heart area. This chakra is the connection between the lower, more primal, energy centres, into the higher centres of higher consciousness.
5. The **Manipura** chakra is located in the solar plexus, just below the navel. The element for this chakra is fire (the fire of digestion). This is our will centre, where we take the desires from the sixth chakra and do them.
6. The **Swadhisthana** chakra is located in the pelvic area and is associated with the water element. It governs our creative juices and the fluidity of life.
7. The **Muladhara** chakra, located at the base of the spine, is associated with the Earth element and governs our most basic primal instincts of survival and the downward flow of energy. Our right to be here, our most primal instincts, come from this Chakra.

This image can make these chakras easier to visualize and understand: [63]

---

[63] "The Seven Chakras for Beginners," *Hands on Health Sheffield*, January 27, 2020, http://www.handsonhealthsheffield.com/holistic_massage/the-seven-chakras-for-beginners/.

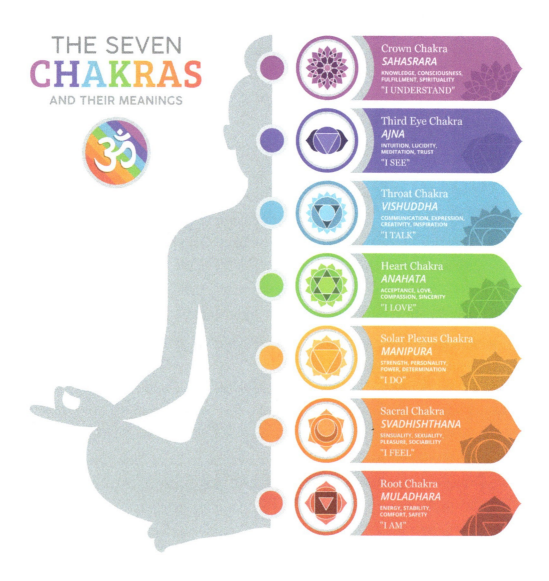

The aim of Laya Yoga is to bring these energy centres into balance, allowing the Kundalini energy to rise from the lower chakra to the higher ones and then transforming that energy to help the individual reach higher consciousness and rid them of their karmic debt.

No one chakra works independently; if one is out of balance, the others must compensate for it. From a Yoga perspective, because we live in the physical realm, we must take care of our survival instincts first. After ensuring our survival, we can focus on higher understanding.

Much like Maslow's Hierarchy of Needs[64], if our most basic needs are not met—safety, food, shelter etc.—we will not grow physically, emotionally, or spiritually. All we are doing at that point is surviving. Take having to go to the bathroom as an example. If you *really* have to go, nothing else matters at that point—not money, not fame. You just have to go!

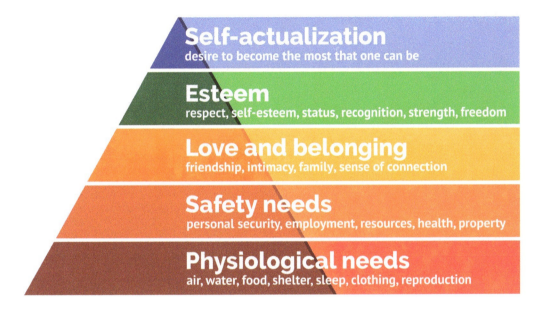

The above pyramid is often thought of as representing the entirety of Maslow's famous hierarchy. Interestingly, Maslow added a new pinnacle to his pyramid

---

64 S. McLeod, "Maslow's Hierarchy of Needs," *Simply Psychology*, December 29, 2020, https://www.simplypsychology.org/maslow.html.

in 1971, which he termed "Transcendence": "Transcendence refers to the very highest and most inclusive or holistic levels of human consciousness, behaving and relating, as ends rather than means, to oneself, to significant others, to human beings in general, to other species, to nature, and to the cosmos."[65]

A more accurate pyramid might look like this[66]:

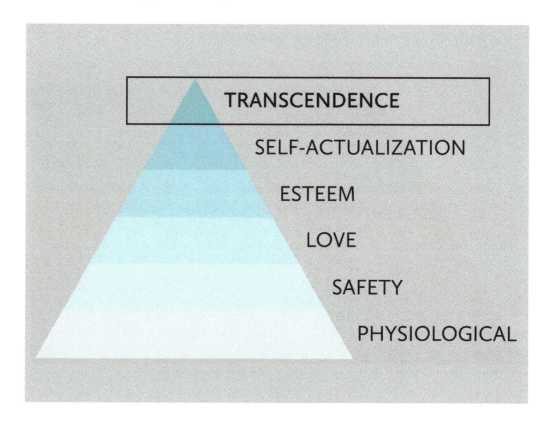

According to Maslow, self-transcendence brings the individual what he termed "peak experiences" in which they transcend their personal concerns and see

---

[65] A.H. Maslow, *The Farther Reaches of Human Nature* (New York, NY: Penguin Books, 1971, 269.),

[66] K. Kowalski, "What is Transcendence? The True Top of Maslow's Hierarchy of Needs," *Sloww*, https://www.sloww.co/transcendence-maslow/.

from a higher perspective. These experiences often bring strong positive emotions, like joy, peace, and a well-developed sense of awareness. Someone who is highly self-transcendent may also experience "plateau experiences" in which they consistently maintain or enter a state of serenity and higher perspective.[67] This is what is experienced when the **Sahasrara** chakra and the associated state of Samādhi (the Eighth Limb of Yoga) is activated.

Yoga has the ability to help you reach this point of transcendence. More immediately important, however, is its ability to take you out of "the darkness." It can help you rebuild the foundation of your life and take you into the higher frequencies of the upper chakras one breath at a time, one asana at a time, one mediation at a time. It only works if you follow the practices faithfully; what you put into it you will get back out. There are many obstacles in Yoga, and removing them takes work. The first one we want to get rid of is the "shitty committee," or that voice that says you can't, you are not enough.

The first step?

Just do it, dammit!

---

[67] J.G. Messerly, "Summary of Maslow on Self-Transcendence," *Reason and Meaning*, January 18, 2017, https://reasonandmeaning.com/2017/01/18/summary-of-maslow-on-self-transcendence/.

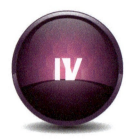

The Darkness

Valuing ourselves is one of the hardest things to do: "... love your neighbor as yourself" (Mark 12:31). The Lord instructed us to love Him above all else and then love our neighbours as we love ourselves. There are no greater commandments than these according to the holy scriptures. But how do we do that when some days we can barely tolerate ourselves? The trials of life and my lack of self-worth have led me to the practice of Yoga, a practice that has been passed down for thousands of years. Along with those treasured verses from the scriptures, the practices of Yoga have not only taught me to love and value myself, but to love and value others. *Maitri*, also called *Metta,* is a Buddhist practice that cultivates compassionate care toward oneself. This practice is simple yet complex at the same time, so I will guide you through it step by step.

1. Sit in a comfortable seated position, either on the floor or in a chair.
2. Close your eyes and begin to focus on your breath.
3. Take a deep inhale and count to six, then exhale and count to six. Do this four times.
4. Allow your breath to settle into a natural rhythm

5. Now shift your attention to the space within your chest, the heart's centre.
6. *To a Loved One:* Recall someone who allows you to feel love, such as a family member or a pet. Hold on to that feeling while you repeat the Mantra below, either out loud or silently:

> May You be Well, May You be Safe, May You be Happy and Healthy
> May You be Peaceful and at Ease
> AMEN

7. *To a Neutral Person:* Now recall a neutral person, an acquaintance for whom you hold neither good nor bad feelings. Repeat the mantra while picturing this person.
8. *To an Enemy:* This is a bit more difficult. Recall someone for whom you hold negative feelings, and again repeat the mantra while picturing them. This can be very difficult to do. The first time I did it, I thought, *No fucking way am I going to send loving thoughts to this person!* But when I allowed myself to do this, it was the most profound experience of my life. I sat there and pictured this person in front of me, and I sent loving kindness to them. I began to cry, but the tears weren't for me. They were for the suffering happening within that person. This is where forgiveness can be very powerful—when we don't forget but we truly do forgive. This frees us from the bondage of the pain we think they created in us.
9. Repeat the mantra to the general public.
10. Repeat the mantra to all sentient beings.
11. Repeat the mantra to the planet.
12. Repeat the mantra to the universe; remember that God reigns over all in equal measure.
13. Repeat the mantra back to yourself.

14. Take a deep breath and sit quietly for a few minutes. The Metta Prayer is one of the most powerful Mantras.

> May *you* be Well, May *you* be Safe, May *you* be Happy and Healthy
> May *you* be Peaceful and at Ease
> AMEN

While to some the thought of loving oneself may seem selfish, the basis of this practice is that once we can truly respect and value our own being, we can give that love to others. This kind of love doesn't mean we disregard the feelings of others to serve the self. It means we take time to care for and nurture our own well-being. I believe that most crimes and acts of violence are committed by people who have little regard for themselves, and ultimately for others. Most of us are taught our self-worth early in life by our caregivers, and if our own parents or caregivers didn't value and love us, then who would? If that's the case, this modelling of parenting creates a void, a vast emptiness that sometimes takes a lifetime to fill back up, if it can be filled at all. If we lack self-worth, as I did, we begin the search outside of ourselves to fill that bottomless pit, to ease the pain we feel inside, and we wait desperately for someone or something to take it away. Some wait a lifetime for someone to love them enough to validate their own self-worth, and some never find that love. This isn't a matter of blaming our parents or our caregivers for our downfalls; it's merely the reality and the result of living with dysfunction and neglect.

That sense of self-worth (or lack thereof) can lead to all kinds of deviant and harmful behaviour, from alcoholism to sexual addictions, drug addictions, work addictions, etc. In rare cases, monsters are just monsters without any obvious reason. I'm not a psychiatrist, so I can't speak for the many different mental disorders that might contribute to deviant behaviour. That being said, I still believe that at the core of it all is a lack of caring, a lack of self-worth and self-caring, an "evil" of the spirit. I believe it's in our nature to be loved and feel loved. We're wired that way, and when we don't feel self-love, then how do we give love to others?

The sad reality is that many children grew up in dysfunctional circumstances and felt unloved and unwanted. I have no doubt that some of you reading this book identify with this feeling. Does that mean you have no value? Not at all! It only means that your parents or caregiver, for reasons beyond your control, didn't know how to give you that value. You can't give something you don't have in you. The good news is that you can start to recover from that lack of self-worth by beginning to love yourself unconditionally. This beautiful Buddhist[68] phrase sums it up: "You as much as anyone else deserves love, compassion and happiness."[69] You just have to do the hard work needed to recover your sense of self-worth; the hard work is well worth the effort.

YOU CAN RECOVER!

Believe you are worth it. I promise you: YOU ARE WORTH IT!

I watched a video recently that showed a father going on a date with his five-year-old daughter.[70] He prepared himself as he would for any first date, groomed and dressed in his finest suit and tie. He knocked at the door on his knees and greeted his little girl. She opened the door and, with a magnificent smile, said, "Hi, Daddy!" He hugged her and told her how beautiful she was, and off they went on their date. What most struck me about the father was that

---

[68] The earliest documented use of a similar phrase comes from Burmese monk Mahasi Sayadaw in Part II of his 1983 booklet, *Brahmavihara Dhamma,* which itself is a translation of canon Buddhist scriptural texts: http://www.buddhanet.net/brahmaviharas/bvd020.htm

[69] Sharon Salzberg included a similar quote in *Lovingkindness: The Revolutionary Art of Happiness* (1995, 31). She presents these words as if they were a quote from the Buddha. Variations of this quote can be found in similar texts, including John Amodeo's *The Authentic Heart: An Eightfold Path to Midlife Love* (2001), and Laura Doyle's *The Surrendered Wife: A Practical Guide for Finding Intimacy, Passion, and Peace with a Man* (2001).

[70] Nonya Business, "The Best First Date," YouTube video, 2:29, June 13, 2014, https://www.youtube.com/watch?v=GiOJuIPl8vE.

he was present and attentive to the needs of his daughter. I thought to myself, *What a wonderful world this would be if all fathers treated their children like that. They would know the meaning of love.* This type of "love" models for children how to love and give love freely without fear. It goes without saying that children need both parents as role models, and it turns out that the role model of the father figure is extremely important to the family structure. I believe that fathers who are physically present can be emotionally detached (absent) from the family structure. As a parent, you have to realize that your children need a role model. They are watching and soaking in *everything you say and do!* It's not an understatement to say that if you screw up as a parent, you will screw up your children. That is a fact! This isn't about blame; blaming is useless and serves no purpose. It's about becoming aware of how our actions affect others, specifically the lives of our children. My son, even at a very young age, would remind me, "My failure as a child is your failure as a parent," and I agree with that statement 100 per cent.

Each of us has the responsibility, regardless of circumstances, to take control of our life and current situation. On the path of Yoga, there are no victims. We use the practice of Yoga to become aware, to remove the veils of ignorance so that we can make better choices that will shift our current situation for the better. We may not be able to change the situation, but we always have the control to shift the way we react to it. One of the best tools on the Path is the practice of meditation, and any practices like Metta.

Growing up, dysfunction in the family was a way of life, passed down from one generation to the next. My parents were both war babies and carried the scars of dysfunction and neglect throughout their lives. My mom married very young to "dad number one," who left her stranded with four children and no means to support herself. She didn't have a home to go to when times were tough, but she did the very best she could, based on the modelling she had received as a child. Home to her was not the image that typically comes to mind when you think of the word "home." *Ozzie and Harriet* and *Leave it to Beaver* were far from the reality of her world growing up. I wish my mom had had a father like the ones in those shows above, but she wasn't so fortunate. Father-deprivation is a more reliable predictor of criminal activity than race, environment, or poverty. Father-deprived children comprise 72 per cent of all teenage murderers, 60 per cent of rapists, and 70 per cent of kids incarcerated. They are twice as likely to quit school and eleven times more likely to be violent. They make up three out of four teen suicides, 80 per cent of the adolescents in psychiatric hospitals, and 90 per cent of runaways.[71]

My mom grew up for the most part in foster care, being bounced from one home to another. Her mother died when she was only seven years old, and her father returned from the war so full of rage that he drowned in alcohol. While in his care, she sadly became the recipient of his inner demons. She never gave specifics of what happened to her as a child, except for being locked in the basement whenever she did something that displeased her dad. The image of a small child huddled in a corner of a cold, dark basement is incomprehensible to most people, and so it should be. For my mom, it was an everyday occurrence. She grew up with all of the scars of a lifetime of abuse and neglect, and sadly passed some of those scars down to her children. When my mom couldn't care for us, she did the only thing she knew to do: leave us in the care of the same system she grew up in. We were bounced from one foster home to another until the day she met the man who would adopt us and raise us as his own.

"Dad number two" grew up in the same situation as my mom did: his mom also died when he was very young, and his dad had even more rage than my grandfather. My dad told me stories of hiding in the woodshed from his father to escape beatings, he left home at the age of 14, back in the day that was not uncommon. He shared one story of working on a local farm, the farmer let him live under the porch, and he fed him onions and lard. And I complained about

---

[71] K. Thomas, "Lost Generation Part 5: Statistics on Father-Deprived Children, *Canadian Association for Equality*, November 25, 2014, https://equalitycanada.com/lost-generation-part-5-statistics-on-father-deprived-children/.

a peanut butter sandwich. When my dad shared that story with me, my heart softened for him, and I could see that little child in him so desperately wanting to be loved and cared for.

And isn't that what we all want? To be loved, to be accepted, to find some peace in our hearts.

One of the many gifts Yoga has given me, is allowing myself to see my parents, not as my parents, but as fellow human beings with their own stories, hurts and personal struggles. I love my parents and understand that they did the very best they knew how at the time. I don't hold any ill feelings toward them, and I don't mean to disrespect them in any way, I do, however, believe that sharing my story will help others to not feel alone and will give them some hope that they too can heal. We can forgive those who have trespassed against us, and we can forgive ourselves for trespassing against others. Don't kid yourself: we all trespass and we all need forgiveness at one point or another.

I believe that we're all just mirrors of each other. When that mirror reflects something negative back to us, our first instinct is to blame others. If the mirror constantly reflects a negative image, the world becomes a lonely and scary place to live in, and that negative feedback reinforces our current reality. The reflection I saw prior to my Yoga practice was an accumulation of a lifetime of Karma. Like putting money in the bank, I and the generations before me had spent more than we had deposited. All human beings want the same thing, no matter what your background or the colour of your skin. We all desire happiness and to be accepted for who and what we are. I felt defeated and very alone, and that loneliness was consuming and destroying not only me but those around me.

The desperation and loneliness I felt affected the way I parented, the way I engaged with my family and with my partner. I was becoming more withdrawn and depressed on the inside, literally dying from the inside out. I kept these feelings of desperation to myself, having learned at a very young age to stuff them deep inside. After all, only weak people show feelings, correct? We teach our young children—especially our boys— not to feel; we say things like "Don't cry, shake it off, don't be such a sissy, don't act like a girl." But what does it mean to not act like a girl? Like being a girl is something to be feared—but that's another topic entirely. All of these messages contribute to the way we interact with the world. Now add some deep generational dysfunction, and you have a recipe for disaster. The problem with stuffing down feelings is that they're like young children—they just keep getting louder until you take the time to listen to them. They may come out in the unhealthiest of ways if we don't. Often, we don't want to feel them, but in order for them to be quiet, we must take that time to listen and *feel*!

Prior to my Yoga practice, I was going through life on an unconscious level, feeling like a victim who had no control over her life. Before I became aware, I too left some long-lasting scars in my children. I was a young mother without the proper skills to give my young children what they needed to grow into healthy adults. The sins of the father and mother become the sins of their sons and daughters. My prayer is that my children can overcome any wrongdoing I passed onto them, and that they can heal for the sake of future generations to come.

We only know what we know, and when the veils of ignorance are lifted, we must do what we can to heal any damage we've done to others along this path of life, otherwise we take that Karmic debt into the next life until we've paid it in full. I think that's why the Christian belief is so alluring. Christ took humanity's sins (our collective Karmic debt) to the cross, and with his blood, washed us clean as snow. That's one heavy burden to bear; I can't fathom the weight he felt on his shoulders while he carried that cross. It's no wonder he cried out, "My God, my God, why hast thou forsaken me?" (Matthew 27:46, KJV; Mark 15:34). That being said, I still think we must take responsibility for our current situation and do what we can to better our life and the lives of all sentient beings on this planet. That belief is at the core of the Yoga tradition; thinking of oneself as a victim is not allowed on the Path of Yoga.

None of us know what will happen after our soul leaves our body. All we can do is take the lessons of this life, learn from them, and not repeat them over and over. After all, the definition of insanity is doing the same thing over and over again but expecting different results.[72] Even with this knowledge, we repeat old patterns. I know I've been guilty of doing just that: "Crap, that burner is still hot!" So perhaps I shouldn't put my hand on the burner any longer if I choose not to get burned.

I was searching for something to fill the void in my soul and heart. I would read self-help books and any spiritual book I could get my hands on. Coles was my favourite store, and the "New Age" section my favourite aisle. I thought, *This book will probably be displayed in New Age*. I read the Bible, books on Buddhism, Zen, and any spiritual book I could find, searching and longing for the answers I was seeking. I would attend church, listen to the sermons, and pray that God would give me the answers to my suffering. Still, I thought to myself, *Where on Earth is this God I've been hearing about?*

I spent a great deal of time during my twenties on my hands and knees praying to God, literally begging to be released from the torture that was going on in my mind and body, most of which I had absolutely no control over. Nothing I did gave me any relief from my inner torment, until the day I went to my first Yoga class. Turns out these books and ancient texts do hold the secrets we need, but until we actually apply the teachings, they're just words on a page. All those positive affirmations that have become the norm mean nothing unless we put their messages into practice.

This was the beginning of my journey, the journey to my Soul and to who I am: I am Yoga! Since that day, I've gone through many transformations, but I have established the rock foundation that I continue to build upon. Jesus said, "Therefore whoever hears these sayings of Mine, and does them, I will liken him to a wise man who built his house on the rock: and the rain descended, the floods came, and the winds blew and beat on that house; and it did not fall, for

---

[72] C. Sterbenz, "12 Famous Quotes That Always Get Misattributed, *Business Insider*, October 7, 2013. https://www.businessinsider.com/misattributed-quotes-2013-10#:~:text=AP%20Photo%20We've%20all,He%20never%20said%20it

it was founded on the rock" (Matthew 7:24–25). The rock of Yoga has helped me through some very painful and difficult times and gave me the tools to face the next few years following the beginning of my journey. My struggles with my past had already been very difficult, to say the least, but my struggles were about to get a whole lot worse.

My belief system, everything I ever thought about life, love, family, and God was about to be challenged. My practice of Yoga was the foundation I needed to heal old wounds and sustain me through what would be some of the hardest years of my life. I use the word Yoga very loosely. For me, it really means my connection to God. As far back as I can remember, God was in my head; I believed there was one, but was he in my heart and soul? Perhaps not. I think he was more like someone to apologize to when I sinned: "Oh, please, God, forgive me for my sins. Please heal the sick, help the poor, and feed the hungry." All of the usual God stuff we expect, and then we become very disappointed when food doesn't fall from the sky, and when our long list of demands goes unmet. After all, if he created the universe, why can't he drop a pizza from the heavens on a whim? We bargain with God, especially when all else fails us. It's a given, at some point or another, that life will fail us, and we will come knocking at God's door. I struggled with these questions, as most people do at one point or another, and one cold January morning I struggled to the depths of my soul. I cried out to God as never before and begged for some sign, something to show me he or she existed, something to show me that this path of Yoga I was on was the right direction to travel.

A few days before I fell to my knees was a beautifully crisp winter day. You know, the ones when the air is crisp and sharp, and the sky is a crystal blue. I was driving to work, looking up at the sky and thanking God for the most recent blessings in my life. Seven weeks prior, we had just celebrated the birth of our first granddaughter. She was a beautiful blue-eyed angel who brought so much joy and happiness to our family. Fast forward seven weeks to Christmas day, and our second grandson, a healthy, beautiful baby boy, is born. A true Christmas miracle. I was overwhelmed with emotions. The birth of my grandchildren was a fresh start. I had lost my mom six months prior from pancreatic cancer; she had been diagnosed in the fall of 2008 and passed away in June of 2009. Before being properly diagnosed she had been sick for two years, suffering from stomach ailments, shoulder pain, and not being able to eat or sleep. She begged doctors to do something but was told that her symptoms were the result of stress, or a pulled muscle, or many other things. She knew all along it was cancer. We took her to various doctors and emergency rooms, having made countless phone calls to doctors to try and get her some answers. It turns out that if you have a perfect heart rate and blood pressure, the doctors' concerns that you may have a serious ailment greatly decline. Its just stress they would tell her, a pulled muscle etc. etc.

In September of 2008, we drove her to the hospital, where she sat in the emergency room for eight hours in excruciating pain, until she couldn't sit any longer. Upon leaving the emergency room, we told the nurse, "She just can't sit any longer." They asked us to just hold on for a few more minutes, and they would do their best to get to her. The nurse kept her word, and my mother was taken into a room within a few minutes. The doctor asked her a few questions and, recognizing some of the symptoms, ordered a CAT scan and some blood work. It was only a short time after that we were all escorted into a room and given the news that she was full of cancer. Hearing the word "cancer" is bad enough, but hearing "fourth stage pancreatic cancer" is a death sentence. Still, we held on to hope—hope that there would be some treatment that would help her. My mom went through said treatment and endured months of brain fog and nausea, but the end result didn't change. For me, my mom's illness was bittersweet; prior to her illness, I had become estranged from her. As a defence mechanism, I'd put up some pretty strong walls. Upon her diagnosis, I had a heart to heart with her, explaining why I'd put some distance between us. Our conversation gave me the opportunity to let go of some old pain I'd been carrying for years. It shouldn't take a diagnosis to bring us to this point of forgiving another, especially our parents, who gave us life. We cannot go back in time and undo anything; we can only move forward. If I could go back, I would tell my mom, she was deeply loved, and that I am so sorry she had to go through any suffering. The arrival of my grandchildren gave me a sense of new life and new hope, but with the imminent death of my mother looming over us, that was about to be shattered.

I was working at my desk on that cool, crisp December morning when an overwhelming feeling of being suffocated suddenly took over my body. I couldn't catch my breath; I remember sitting there trying to take big breaths and just not being able to get enough air into my lungs. I took a break from my desk and went to the lunchroom to make a tea, but the suffocating feeling wouldn't let up. I was an ex-smoker, so I chalked it up to the damage I'd done to my lungs via twenty years of smoking. Upon returning to my office, I heard a knock at the door, and I opened it to look upon a mutual co-worker of my husband and son, Marc. This co-worker was also a firefighter who had responded to a 911 call at my son's residence. He said, "Your granddaughter has been taken by ambulance to the hospital, with no vital signs."

I remember thinking, *Well, she's at the hospital, so they'll be able to do something*. It didn't register that she had already passed. I was frozen in that moment, and some days I still feel frozen there. I arrived at the hospital a few minutes later to greet my son and daughter-in-law in a room full of nurses and doctors, whose expressions are forever etched in my mind. My granddaughter lay still on a hospital table, cold and lifeless in another room. The attempts to resuscitate her had failed. She was gone. Sudden Infant Death: a healthy child suddenly stops breathing, and the life force within her leaves her body with no rhyme or reason. That day changed the lives of everyone in my family. The pain of watching my son and daughter in law anguishing over the death of their child was absolutely unbearable. To feel so hopeless knowing there are no words that will lesson their pain. The breathlessness I was feeling earlier in my office, I believe, was my connection to my son and his grief upon receiving the news of her death. Life is not predictable; we never know from one moment to the next what's around the corner. *Bad things like this don't happen to us*, I thought, *they happen to other people.*

Wrong.

In my grief, I reached out once again to God. On my mat that January morning, I surrendered with every ounce of my being. I was broken—heart, mind, spirit, all completely shattered. There was nowhere to go but up.

It has been over a decade since that day, the day that changed my life and my family's lives forever. I look at life now as the time before 2009 and the time after. So, what do we do when tragedy happens? Well, it either consumes us or we rise above it! I am forever grateful for the blessing that our little Angel gave us; her seven short weeks on this Earth touched the hearts of many, and those crystal blue eyes that stared into your soul held the mysteries of the universe. I believe she is with my family and I each step of the way through our journeys in life.

I had reached out to God many times before, but this time was very different; there was a desperation I had never experienced before, and I hope I never experience it again. I begged for a sign that I was on the right path. What did he want from me, this God? What direction was I to go in? That evening, I had the most magnificent vision: I dreamt of a courtyard, and in the middle of the courtyard was a fountain. I saw a gentleman dressed in a long gown, and in his hand, he held a statue of a woman with large breasts. In the background was a temple, old and covered in small mosaic tiles that were thousands of different colours. I could hear a chanting sound and music playing. The tiles of the temple clapped in unison with the chanting. When I awoke, I had a feeling of peace and clarity. I knew what I had to do: dive into my Yoga practice and studies.

I worked full-time as a bookkeeper and wondered how I'd be able to pursue this Yoga path while still earning a living. It only took me minutes to locate who was to become my mediation teacher. I found a website called *Towards Stillness Meditation*[73] and saw they offered a Mediation Facilitator training course. But I was still working full-time. I took a chance and emailed the teacher, asking if

---

[73] http://towardstillness.com/

he did any distance education training. He said he would have to consider that, and within a few weeks I was enrolled in his course. I was able to work around my full-time hours, attend the classes on weekends, and learn one on one via Skype—you have to love modern technology. Every step of my Yoga practice has literally unfolded before me: teachers appeared when needed, places to teach appeared, and classes filled up. I am grateful to God, my teachers, and my students for providing me with the lessons I needed to grow on this path.

At a time in my life when I felt defeated and broken, my path of life opened up for me. This in no way diminished the suffering and grief I was feeling. It did, however, give me a sense of hope and a direction to channel my grief and pain. Life can be painful, unpredictable, and downright sad, but it can also be beautiful, unpredictable, and downright glorious. My practice continues to be my rock, the foundation upon which I build my life. It has taught me to realize that life is fragile but also full of magic at the same time. No matter what your story, Yoga can help you overcome old negative patterns and help you live a fuller, happier, and healthier life!

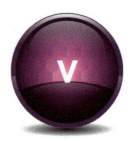

Where Your Journey Begins

*In the words of Pema Chödrön,
"Start Where You Are"*[74]

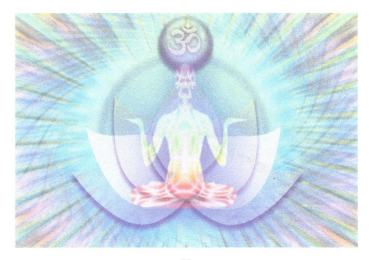

[75]

---

[74] P. Chödrön, *Start Where You Are: A Guide to Compassionate Living.* (Berkeley, CA: Shambala, 2018).

[75] Chakra Wallpaper. *Wallpaper Safari*, January 3, 2018.

Knowing where to start Yoga can be scary and overwhelming. Like the chakras, no Yoga works independently from the others. They all overlap, and you can navigate through them until you find the one that works best for you. Whatever path of Yoga *you* choose, they all aim for the same goal: to reach higher consciousness and realize the true nature of the self, which is ATMAN!

What does this mean in terms of your daily practice? In order for this body to have an expression of the soul, it needs to be healthy. Prevention is always better, but recovery is also possible with proper treatment and in conjunction with the proper Yoga practice that works for each individual. The best advice I can give is to start where you are! As much as Yoga is a means to an end, try to just think about the present. What can you do right this minute to start? Find a Yoga studio near you, search the web for an online Yoga class, reach out and keep reaching until you find a teacher or class that works for you. If you live in a remote area and don't have access to the internet, there are some good books that can help you get started. In addition to the books referenced in this text, I have compiled some resources that I hope you find helpful.

Daily Recommendations

The trick is to start off slow and steady. Build upon a regular routine of small increments by finding what you love and sticking to it! Please remember that you shouldn't do anything that feels uncomfortable, and equally important is that you work at your own pace. What works for me may not work for you. Below is just a general guideline. Please seek out a qualified teacher who can provide you with a routine that works for your specific needs.

1. Your body needs rest, proper food, and exercise.
2. Your mind needs stimulation via learning.
3. Practise mediation to still restless thoughts and change conditioned bad habits.
4. Practise breathing exercises to get the energy properly flowing through your body.

Yoga has become a *big* industry, so it can be difficult to find a type that works for you. You may feel the pressure to fit into the "role" of what a Yogi looks like. When choosing a teacher— which I truly believe we all need, especially at the beginning of our journey—you'll know intuitively if you're a fit. You may consider yourself lucky if you find a teacher who covers all aspects of Yoga: mind, body, breath, and the deeper dimensions of practice. If at first you don't find the one that resonates with you, keep looking until you do. It will be worth it.

You'll find on the journey of Yoga that changing old patterns isn't easy, but it can be done with patience and perseverance. Most importantly, changing a bad habit requires practice, and lots of it! If at first you don't succeed, try and try again. There are many obstacles along this path of Yoga, and one is laziness. There's no room for laziness in our practice, but this doesn't mean we need to do hours of Yoga. We just need to make an intention every day to make Yoga a part of our day-to-day lives. Yes, I know what you're thinking, because I've heard it many times: "I don't have time to do Yoga!" I call bullshit on that. You make time.

Just do it, dammit!

That's the only way to make progress, even if it starts with awareness of one small breath. In fact, we can start there. The Buddhist monk Thich Nhat Hanh offers up this practice to find stillness in the mind:

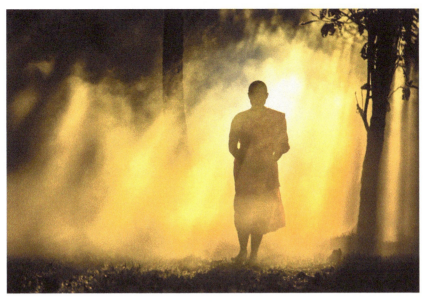

76

"Our breathing is a stable solid ground that we can take refuge in. Regardless of our internal weather—our thoughts, emotions, and perceptions our breathing is always with us like a faithful friend. Whenever we feel carried away, or sunken in a deep emotion, or scattered in worries and projects, we return to our breathing to collect and anchor our mind."

"We feel the flow of air coming in and going out of our nose. We feel how light and natural, how calm and peaceful our breathing functions. At any time, while we are walking, gardening, or typing, we can return to this peaceful source of life.

"We may like to recite:

"'Breathing in I know that I am breathing in.

"'Breathing out I know that I am breathing out.'

---

76   Image source – Adobe Stock

"We do not need to control our breath. Feel the breath as it is. It may be long or short, deep or shallow. With our awareness it will naturally become slower and deeper. Conscious breathing is the key to uniting body and mind and bringing the energy of mindfulness into each moment of our life".[77]

Square Breathing

Breathing is a process that happens on its own without our effort as part of the Autonomic Nervous System, which controls respiration, heart rate, blood pressure, and our fight or flight response. With Yoga you can override this process and take ourselves from the fight or flight to the parasympathetic nervous system, which brings us to a calm state. From here, we can rest and restore. This technique can have a profound calming effect on our minds and bodies. The breathing process has four components:

1. *Puraka* (Inhalation)
2. *Antara Kumbhaka* (Breath Retention After Inhalation)
3. *Rechaka* (Exhalation)
4. *Bahya Kumbhaka* (Breath Retention After Exhalation)

Process

1. Find a comfortable sitting position with a straight spine
2. If you are very tired, lie down with your head supported with a block, bolsters, or cushion.
3. Begin by closing your eyes lightly and start listening to the sounds you hear around you. Often, we try and close out the sounds—which is a practice in itself—but for now, just listen.

---

[77] "Breathing," *Joyful Garden Sangha*, https://www.joyfulgarden.sg/mindfulness/.

4. Begin to take deeper breaths into the abdomen, slow deep, soundless, and long.
5. Now inhale and count to four as you do so.
6. Gently hold this breath and count to four.
7. Exhale and count to four as you do so.
8. Repeat this process for ten rounds
9. Sit quietly for a few minutes and enjoy the calmness cultivated in your body and mind.

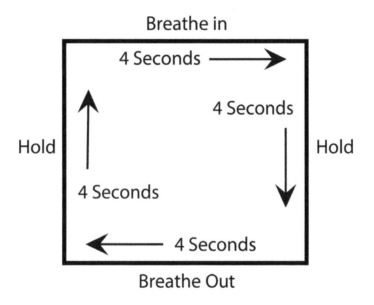

[78]

This may be difficult at first if you're used to upper chest breathing, so be gentle with the process. Yoga and its practices are not quick fixes but a change in our

---

[78] M. Eichenseer, "The Life Hack You Can Take Anywhere: Breathing, *Medium*, June 28, 2016, https://mikenseer.medium.com/the-life-hack-you-can-take-anywhere-breathing-20f0627d0f73

habits over time. If you want to change the course of your life, you have to begin to take a new path, and this starts with awareness. Awareness starts with breath! Awareness is the key to change; if we're not aware of our daily habits, we can't change them. Much of what we do is on an unconscious level; belief systems that have been ingrained into us over the course of our lives rule our every action. Karma is action: change the thought, change the action; change the habits, change our destiny.

From Mind to Body

Once you've found some stillness in your breath, it's time to find strength in the body.

I speculate that at one point there may have been as many as 108,000 poses.[79] This has been reduced to 84,000, of which we mostly use about 84.[80] For daily practice, finding two or three to work with on a regular basis and building on that would be most realistic and beneficial.

> The prerequisites of all Yoga are morality, a spiritual disposition, and regular practice of Yogic exercises. One form of Yoga, Hatha Yoga, gives first attention to the physical body, which is the vehicle of the spirit's existence and activity. Purity of the mind is not possible without purity of the body in which it functions, and by which it is affected.[81]

---

[79] H. Avery, "108: Yoga's Sacred Number," *Wanderlust*, https://wanderlust.com/journal/108-yogas-sacred-number/.

[80] D. Garrigues, "84,000 postures and Krishnamacharya," *David Garrigues*, 2021, https://davidgarrigues.com/writings/84000-postures-and-krishnamacharya.

[81] S.V. Devananda, *The Complete Illustrated Book of Yoga.* (New York, NY: Three Rivers Press, 1995), 13.

Remember, Yoga is about uniting. If your body isn't strong, such as when you're hungry or tired, you're less likely to do Yoga. If you carve out some time in the morning (about ten minutes to start with) to do simple poses, you'll begin to build strength and confidence.

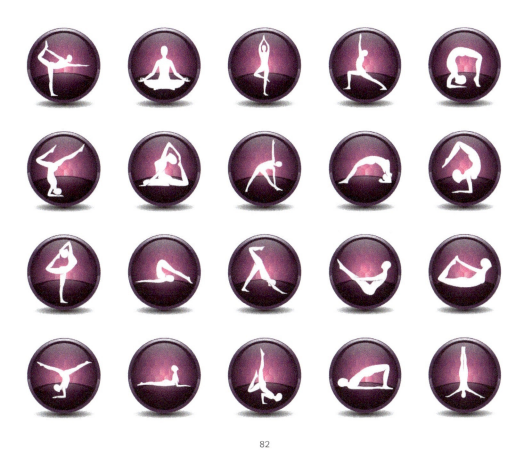

82

When it comes to your asana (pose) practice, it can be hard to know where to start. Here is a nice morning routine you can try, and you can build on it if it works for you. Starting out with ten minutes of Relaxation Yoga, or *Yoga Nidra*,

---

82   Image source – Adobe Stock

is a fantastic way to begin any day. Yes, you just woke up and washed your face, and now it's time to relax the body and prepare for the day. If you ask anyone who attends a Yoga class, they'll tell you that *Savasana* (corpse pose) is the pose they love the most. It was the one that hooked me, and I haven't looked back since. It allows the body time to come out of fight or flight mode and reach a place of deep relaxation. In *Yoga Nidra*, you leave your waking state, go through a dreaming state, and then into a deep, sleep-like state, yet you remain fully awake.

Process

1. Start off in *Savasana* (lying on your back with head supported by a small cushion or folded blanket, arms out to the side with the palms facing up, legs comfortably apart).
2. Close your eyes and form a clear intention.
3. Take a few deep breaths, emphasizing exhalation.
4. Starting with your right side, rotate your awareness through all parts of the body—limb by limb—in quick succession.
5. Become aware of each finger, the palms of your hands, the back of your hands, and each of your hands as a whole.
6. Become aware of your forearms, elbows, upper arms, shoulder joints, shoulders, and neck.
7. Become aware of each section of your face (forehead, eyes, nose, lips, and so on) in turn.
8. Become aware of your ears and scalp and move your awareness down to your throat.
9. Become aware of your shoulder blades, your chest, and rib cage.
10. Become aware of your stomach, lower abdomen, and waist.
11. Become aware of whole spine, down to your buttocks and genitalia.
12. Become aware of your thighs, the top and back of your knees, your shins and calves.

13. Become aware of your ankles, the tops of your feet, your heels and soles.
14. Become aware of each toe in turn, and each foot as a whole.
15. Be aware of your body as a whole.
16. Repeat the process until adequate depth of relaxation is achieved, always ending with whole-body awareness.
17. Be aware of your whole body and the space surrounding it.
18. Feel the stillness and peace and reaffirm your initial intention.
19. Mentally prepare to return to ordinary consciousness.
20. Gently move your fingers for a few moments, take a deep breath, and then open your eyes.

"The Bodhisattva-mahasattva sees both the evil elephant and the evil friend as one and not two. Why so? Because both destroy one's own self. The Bodhisattva never fears the evil elephant, but fears the evil friend. Why? The evil elephant only harms the body, not the mind. The evil friend destroys both."[83]

Transitioning from Being Conscious to Being Awake: A Morning Asana Routine

Sun Salutations (Sanskrit: *Surya Namaskar*) is a sequence of twelve postures. The sun is the source of all life and energy on our planet, including us. No sun means no life. This practice is a way to respect and appreciate the life-giving energy the sun provides, and at the same time strengthen the body by keeping the spine supple and strong. In the practice of Hatha Yoga as well as other types of Yoga, it's commonly agreed that there are two energy channels that flow along either side of the spine and cross over a third, main channel. The main channel

---

[83] K. Yamamoto, *The Mahayana Mahaparinirvana Sūtra.* Translated into English from Dharmakshema's Chinese version in Taisho Tripitaka, (1973), Vol. 12, No. 374, 307. http://lirs.ru/do/Mahaparinirvana_Sutra,Yamamoto,Page,2007.pdf

that flows along the centre of the spine is called the *Sushumna,* while the left and right channels are called the *Ida* and *Pingala,* or Sun and Moon. The Ida flows up the left side and represents the cool feminine aspect. Its opposite, the Pingala, runs up the right and represents the hot male aspect.

We won't dive too deeply into the philosophy of these teachings. For now, it's enough to simply practise Sun Salutations. As you move through the sequence below, it's important to focus on breathing. Remember, awareness starts with breath! Inhale as you extend or raise your arms overhead, and exhale as you flex or fold. Always begin with the breath and then follow through with the corresponding movement. You can start with a few rounds and work your way up to twelve rounds in the morning. If you want to slow the practice down, you can hold each posture for up to five square breaths. Advanced practitioners may choose to increase the inhale and exhale to a comfortable length, as long as the exhale equals or exceeds the inhale without strain.

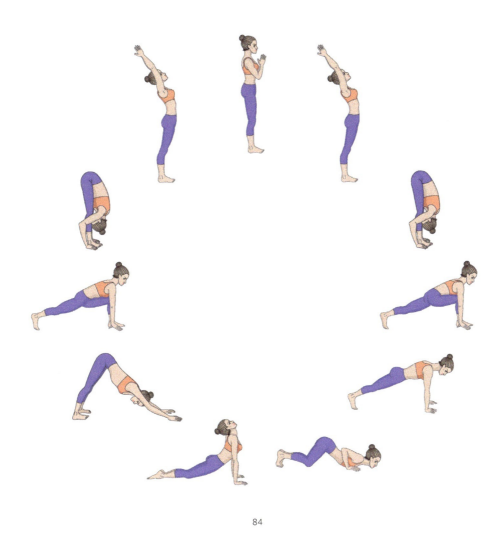

84

When you have completed your desired rounds of Sun Salutations, you can once again return to *Savasana* to complete your morning practice.

There are as many variations of these practices as there are people on the planet. When it comes to your personal practice, it's best to listen to how you feel prior to the practice and afterwards. If you're feeling exhausted afterwards,

---

84   Image source – Adobe Stock

this is an indication that your practice needs to be adjusted. Meeting with a qualified teacher can help you determine your personal needs. The practice I have suggested is simply a starting point to build upon.

We now have our internal energy flowing with pranayama, and the body is energized with our asana practice.

Next we need to turn our attention to the mind! It does have a mind of its own, doesn't it? Remember that according to Patañjali, Yoga is the stilling of the fluctuations of the mind: the thought waves that control our behaviour.

When it comes to starting meditation practices, one can become very overwhelmed. How can we measure ourselves against the Buddhas and the Christs of the world? Where you start will be different from where I started, as we all have different experiences and life challenges. One thing that is the same for all of us, however, is breathing. Without breathing, we cannot live. Breath anchors us to this life, and it's this foundation that Yoga practices and meditations are built from. As you settle back into your meditation position on your mat, with body stretched and energy flowing, begin to bring your attention back to your breath. Remember the words of Thich Nhat Hanh:

> "Breathing in I know that I am breathing in.
> Breathing out I know that I am breathing out."

Try to focus on this for three to five minutes. As your meditational focus improves, you can increase this to ten minutes, fifteen minutes, and then as long as you can comfortably sit in a calm, peaceful state.

These practices are a solid base for developing and building upon daily meditation practices, and they're an excellent place to start your Yoga journey. I advise you to seek the help of a qualified teacher when you're ready for more advanced practices.

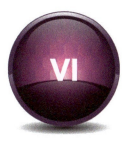

Returning to the Light

Before I discovered Yoga, I was in the "darkness" on all levels of my being. My body was a wreck, my emotions were all over the map, and my energy was nonexistent. Getting out of bed became a struggle most days; it was so much easier to hide under the covers and ignore the world entirely. Each morning I awoke with a deep sense of dread that showed no signs of fading away. It took a great deal of mental and physical strength to drag my ass out of bed, and most people who knew me were clueless when it came to my suffering. Externally, I had become very good at faking how I felt; my carefully crafted social mask showed no signs of anger, frustration, resentment, or, especially, fear—fear that I would be found out and called a fraud for pretending I had my life together. What a joke it is that we suffer in silence for fear of being judged, when we all judge one another just the same. For so many, the voices of others in our heads have become our biggest enemy: the voice of a caregiver calling you stupid, a teacher mocking your misspelling of the word "essay" and having you write it on the board every day for the rest of the year, your internal voice, whose ugly truths only you can hear. These are the used furniture in the basement of your mind, buried beneath the shiny floorboards in your mental living room. As with all things buried in the basement, this used furniture accumulates dust, drawing you in and awaiting the opportunity to bury you down there alongside it. We must take the time to clean up that old furniture, to shake off the dust and replace it with something new. It's our job to look after our own well-being, and it can't be made into anyone else's responsibility. I know it sounds harsh, but bad shit does—no, *will*—happen. That's just the reality of life. When we begin the hard work of self-study, we begin to look at ourselves and others in a new light.

This doesn't mean we no longer need any help—we are human and always will—but it *does* mean that you're the only one who knows what you need. If you don't know, how on Earth can you expect another person to know? This doesn't mean that we disregard the feelings and needs of others in our lives, for we all play many roles in this life, and each one has its own important responsibilities. This is what makes the world go 'round; if all we cared about was ourselves, there would be no need for anyone in our lives, right? Self-care is not selfish. What *is* selfish is meeting our own personal needs with no regard for how it affects others around us. How do you practise this selfless form of self-care? You get proper sleep, eat and exercise properly, have clothes and a shelter, and actively live your life's purpose. Selfish behaviour is more like cranking the stereo at 3:00 a.m. because you want to listen to your favourite tunes while others are trying to sleep. If you follow the Eight Limbs of Yoga, you will naturally realize that what you do affects others. With non-harm being first and foremost of the limbs, everything else naturally falls into place.

Self-care and its natural extension, *self-love,* do not involve giving up your responsibilities to your family, friends, and society in general. Rather, it's the practice of strengthening—or rebuilding, if necessary—your own sense of identity. As humans, we have similar traits, and we all breathe the same air. However, we have also been gifted individual likes and dislikes and unique personalities that make each person a miracle in and of themselves. The bottom line is that the voices of others need to be plucked out of the basements of our minds; to do this, we must learn to practise self-care.

My personal journey out of the darkness started with my very first Yoga class on a Monday night at 7:30 p.m. That a Yoga class was even being offered in my rural, conservative little town was a miracle in and of itself. I thought to myself, *I am in!* There was nothing particularly fancy about the room, but it was clear that the teacher had taken great care in preparing the space with intention and love. She had a small CD player, and as she prepared the music for the class, it was clear that she was preparing herself as well, both mentally and emotionally. I was impressed by her calm demeanour and calming presence. When the class started, I was unsure what to expect, but it flowed exceptionally smoothly—from a warm-up to breathing practices, to asana practices, and then what we come to Yoga for … the relaxation at the end. What stuck in my mind were her words: "This time is just for you." I had never in my life taken time "just for me." I was hooked and have never looked back. She spoke this weird language that captivated my attention; I learned later it was the language of Yoga: Sanskrit.

I also learned that I was not in particularly good physical shape; my years of not looking after my body had finally caught up with me. Standing in warrior pose that first class I thought my legs were going to give out on me, but I held my stance strong and tall regardless. I love the warrior sequence because it gives me a feeling of inner power, even if my body tells me otherwise; it's my edge. In Yoga we don't want to push ourselves to the point of exhaustion, but we want to find our edge, that place where we feel the heat of *tapas*, where we feel the shake in our legs, where we dig deep into our mental capacity and hold our ground, even if only for one more breath.

One of my classes in India stands out to me. The teacher, Mohan Yogi, would guide us into a chair pose that can be incredibly challenging. He would keep us there for what seemed like forever but was probably just ten breaths or so. At about the time we would all start to sink down, he would say "up, up, up!" All of a sudden, you could see the room full of students stand just a bit taller in the pose. "The body follows the mind," he would say.

I would also argue that the body controls the mind! Either way, the discipline of Yoga demands that we work with this communication from mind to body and body to mind. Most often, we only hear that communication when the body and mind are screaming at each other in pain or suffering. Yoga allows us the space to listen, to bridge this gap. We can then take steps to correct what is out of balance. In my case, my body was screaming, and my emotional state was well beyond a scream. It had sought shelter within me and became the internal silence of my soul shutting down.

I used to believe that we are all born with a soul and that it doesn't change throughout our lives. I would now argue that our soul can be diminished by life's trials and tribulations. But it can also be elevated by our will to live a happy, healthy life. When you're living your life's purpose, your soul is content. This is where Karma comes along: if we diminish the soul in this life, it needs another life to regain what it lost, but it carries with it the unresolved issues and feelings from each life. In a sense, it's our responsibility to clean up the crap we may have been born into and then do our best not to contribute to passing that along into the next body it's born into. In the end, we have to make a conscious shift from thinking that life is haphazard and that we are not the creators of our own lives. When we make the shift to go within to that stillness, we tap into the Gap, which Deepak Chopra says is "filled with pure potentiality,"[85] and is where all things are possible. But we have to do the hard work of becoming aware in the moment. And do not kid yourself: this is very hard work. It takes courage to be a spiritual warrior, to wake up from your conditioned responses and live a life of intention and attention.

How are you going to start your own journey out of the darkness? It only takes one breath of awareness, one moment of closing your eyes and listening, to start your journey!

Not all Yoga focuses on the profound connection of the mind, body, and breath. Some studios only focus on the physical part of Yoga, and while this isn't "bad" or "wrong," I strongly feel that Yoga practices should include all three

---

[85] D. Chopra, *The Seven Spiritual Laws of Success*, 1994, 7, https://taxuna.files.wordpress.com/2015/11/deepak-chopra-the-7-laws-of-success.pdf.

dimensions: asana practice to strengthen the body, breathing practices to keep the energies balanced, and meditation practices to discipline the mind.

Right now, wherever you are, take a moment to stop and listen, *really* listen. What do you hear? How many noises can you identify? Are they pleasant? Unpleasant? In this moment, it doesn't matter. Just *listen*. Now, take a deep breath. Another. Another. With each breath, slow down the speed of your exhalation just a bit.

Now, close your eyes, if it's safe to do so, and listen again. Now what do you hear? Congratulations, you have started your journey toward being aware! It's that simple yet complex at the same time!

I left that class feeling like I had just found the pot of gold at the end of the rainbow and unlocked the secrets of the universe. I continued to attend weekly classes, two if I could manage, and I could feel a change happening within me. This had actually not been my first Yoga experience; I had tried a class a few years prior this one. It was fantastic, but I now know that it only focused on the asana portion of the practice. I am so grateful for the Monday night town hall Yoga class that changed my life and set me on a path of no return.

I get to live this life every day, spreading the healing benefits of this ancient practice.

How blessed am I?

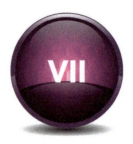

My Sādhanā

Sādhanā is your personal practice that works specifically for your constitution and personal needs. It may change from day to day. The word Sādhanā translates to "practice, of self-transformation."[86] Jaggi Vasudev, better known as Sadhguru, defines Sādhanā as follows:

> Everything can be Sādhanā. The way you eat, the way you sit, the way you stand, the way you breathe, the way you conduct your body, mind and your energies and emotions – this is Sādhanā. Sādhanā does not mean any specific kind of activity, Sādhanā means you are using everything as a tool for your wellbeing.[87]

When we go to the mat, it's the perfect opportunity to practise self-awareness. It's a time to reflect and pay attention to what your body is trying to communicate

---

[86] O. Swami, "The Four Pillars of Sādhanā," *Om Swami*, December 22, 2011, https://os.me/the-four-pillars-of-sadhana/.

[87] J. Vasudev, "The What & Why of Sādhanā," *Official Website of Sadhguru, Isha Foundation*, December 6, 2012, https://isha.sadhguru.org/ca/en/wisdom/article/the-what-why-of-sadhana.

to you today. I believe your body is actually much more intelligent than your mind. It would need to be, otherwise it wouldn't be able to survive the attacks it faces every day from what we eat and how we interact with the environment around it. If we don't pause to pay attention, we may not catch the cues it's giving us until it's too late.

I recently purchased a Fitbit®, which tells me when I need to get up, move around, etc. They're great, but they only detect movement. They don't measure your amount of proper rest, your stress levels, or your breath respiration ... at least not yet. On the other hand, our bodies have the ability to know what they need for their optimal health if we just tune into them.

Tuning in is the first step.

When I notice I feel very tense during my practice, it's an opportunity for me to do more stretches to release the tension. While this seems like it would be an easy-peasy thing to do, my mind says: *Time to do the dishes, the laundry, check your email...* When this freaking list seems unending, I must remember to go back to my breath and my body, back to the present moment. The practice of Yoga is making a conscious effort to come back—time and time and time again—to your breathing in the present moment. With practice, this will transcend your awareness, and you'll be able to do so subconsciously. This is the true essence of Yoga that the Rishis were trying to teach us, handed down from the heavens to assist us in this life experience.[88]

Our modern-day world is rife with capitalism and consumerism, constantly reinforcing the value of "things." We are always grasping for more, and more, and more, and it's just never enough. It's truly the grandest illusion to think that these things are meaningful. Nothing in this world is permanent; it is ever-changing and evolving, just as we are as people. Think about the times in your life when you were completely present in the moment. The last time was

---

[88] H. Scharfe, "Education in India," from *Handbook of Oriental Studies, Volume 2: South Asia* (The Netherlands: Brill, 2002), 13-15.

probably a birth, a wedding, or a death. Those times bring us into the present, mostly because we're paying attention. I can describe the entire day my granddaughter died: the smell in the air, the colour of the sky, the crispness of that winter day. I can walk through that day from the time I got up in the morning until I cried myself to sleep that night with an anguish I wish never to feel again. This kind of pain is sadly a natural part of life, as is the beauty of birth. Just as sunrise must be followed by sunset, birth must be followed by death. So goes the cycle of life. The time of our death is not known to us, and most live their lives in denial of the truth that death will come for them too. We may fear death, but we fear *truly living* most of all!

Your daily practice, or Sādhanā, can help you be present in the moment, as well as help you build a strong body and mind. This can include any of the practices described in the previous chapter, should you decide to do them daily. Another way to begin a daily routine is through the simple practice of chanting *om*. Remember that according to the Patañjali Sūtras, *om* is a sacred chant that represents the cycle of birth, life, and death found in nature. It's the source of everything and to which everything will eventually return. The energies that shape our world and all of existence may change form, but they do not disappear. In fact, this is the first law of thermodynamics: energy can be transformed from one form to another but can be neither created nor destroyed.[89] This is referred to as "the law of conservation of energy," and although it's a scientific concept, its spiritual consequences are profound. If energy can be neither created nor destroyed, the same is true of our own energies. In spiritual terms, we don't cease to exist upon death; the energy that constitutes our "selves" simply takes

---

[89] R. Feynman, *The Feynman Lectures on Physics, Volume 1.* (Boston, MA: Addison Wesley, 1970) The particular chapter in question, "Conservation of Energy," is published online at https://www.feynmanlectures.caltech.edu/I_04.html.

on a different form, since we have *always existed* in one form or another and *always will*.[90]

So you will live again. But the question remains, what will you do with *this* life? We so often fear what others will think of us, or that love will be withheld from us as a consequence of pursuing our life's calling. We are bound to this fear of losing love, yet we know that true love allows for the growth and expression of other human beings. To find our life's calling, we need only take the time to stop and listen to the inner voice of wisdom that exists within all of us. Doing this act of self-inquiry regularly is necessary in order to live a life of true purpose.

As I write this chapter, the world is in the midst of the Coronavirus (COVID-19) pandemic. Much of the world is at a standstill—and sometimes seems to have stopped altogether—with no sign of returning to a semblance of normalcy in the future. I think to myself now, as we are confined to our homes and social interaction is limited, *What if I had listened to my fears and talked myself out of taking a trip to India?* I am currently in my sixtieth year on this planet, and in its present disease-ridden state, I likely wouldn't be able to travel. I would have missed out on an amazing experience—one that may very well come to be a once-in-a-lifetime experience—had I not gone to India. I had so many questions for the many devout monks and seasoned yogis there. Through my Sādhanā in India, I found the answers to my questions on my mat as I closed my eyes and drew my attention to the silence within.

Travelling to India was scary. There were many parts I did not look forward to, such as the seventeen-hour plane ride, being gone from home for a month, the financial burden the trip placed on me, etc. But in the end, it was the best thing I'd ever done for myself. It cost me a month's wages, plane fare, and

---

[90] To put it scientifically, "a consequence of the law of conservation of energy is that a perpetual motion machine of the first kind cannot exist, that is to say, no system without an external energy supply can deliver an unlimited amount of energy to its surroundings." Found in M. Planck, *Treatise on Thermodynamics* (3rd Ed., A. Ogg, Trans.) (London: Longmans, Green & Co., 1927), 40.

missing my family and friends terribly. But I gained the knowledge that I can overcome my fears, I can evolve, I can meet new challenges with courage. This, as a friend put it, was my rite of passage. I've had many obstacles to overcome, and you have in your life too. They are opportunities for us to dig deep, to either overcome or sometimes simply accept that we don't have control over anything.

Your Sādhanā will be the hardest part of this journey. At first there's an exciting feeling that comes with doing Yoga, so you show up every day on the mat with the feeling you get when you go out on a date for the first time: that feeling of anticipation, joy, and contentment. At first, it was extremely easy for me to carve a daily Yoga practice into my schedule; it was something new and it felt good to take time for myself, which I did faithfully every day for years! Eventually, like all things new, this feeling wears off after a time. At some point, life takes over, the excitement of Yoga being "new" wears off, and it becomes just another thing on your to-do list. When you hit this point, where it becomes mundane and almost bothersome, the real work begins. This is when you start to dig deeper into the practice.

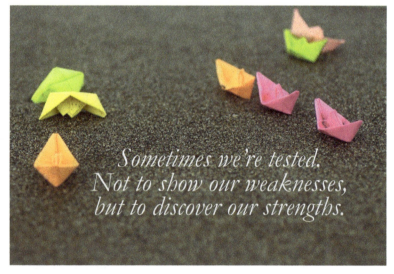

[91]

---

[91] Image source – Adobe Stock

This is where I truly found peace. As with any relationship, your relationship to Yoga takes dedication, perseverance, and the act of showing up every single day. Each of us comes to the mat for a different reason, and each day we show up, the mat presents itself differently as well. When you slow down long enough, you'll notice the aches and pains, the intrusive thoughts, the emotions that we bury in our work, and addictive patterns to avoid. So where does this leave us? On the mat, vulnerable and present! For you, the "mat" can be a chair, a bed, or simply a conscious awareness of your breath.

Over time, your physical ability to perform asanas will evolve, and *you* will evolve. But for this to be the case, you must create a Sādhanā that works for you. It may change from one day to the next, but stick with it, especially when you want to quit. This is where you'll develop your inner strength, and that inner strength will guide you in times of struggle.

We know that the word Yoga means to bring together all aspects of the self into unity. Therefore, we could conclude that your Sādhanā should consist of things that will nurture all aspects of yourself. I can't say this enough: each time you practise your Sādhanā, you build upon the next time you do it! Your daily Sādhanā should include physical movements, prayers, breathing practices, and mindfulness practices such as meditation. It should also transform you off the mat, and those qualities of practice should become part of your daily life.

> Your postures should strengthen your body.
> Your prayers should strengthen your soul.
> Your breathing practices should strengthen your emotions and energy.
> Your meditations should cleanse and strengthen your mind.

One of the biggest challenges you will face in implementing a Sādhanā is getting out of your own head; it begins with believing you can do this and that you are worth the effort. Remember,

Your beliefs become your thoughts, your thoughts become your words, your words become your actions, your actions become your habits, your habits become your values, and your values become your destiny.

Even if you've started a thousand times before, start and keep starting. I know what those voices in your head sound like. They may not be saying the same words as the ones in my head, but the underlying fear is the same: *You can't do this. You will fail again. You are not worthy of succeeding, never mind being worthy of love!* I promise you that you most definitely are worth it. When those voices surface, listen to them, let them have space to clear, give them a gentle smile, and let them fade away as you begin your new journey toward healing.

No one promised you a rose garden, but the most beautiful flowers grow from shit. If you want something bad enough, what are you waiting for? Go after it! Follow your bliss! Follow the yellow brick road! Get off your ass and do it! Yes, you will certainly have challenges. It's what you do with those challenges that determines your future. What you do today builds your tomorrow. So what are you going to do today? Where do you see yourself in ten years? In twenty years? These are not just empty words or fluffy affirmations; these are questions that actually require a great deal of self-study if they're considered seriously. In order to find the true answers to these questions, or to answer them in a way that aligns with your goals in this life, you have to:

Just do it, dammit!

I wish you best of luck with your journey!

Audrey O'Marra

Works Cited

Abbott, G.B. (2014). "The 5 Kinds of Modifications of the Mind." *Original Christianity and Original Yoga.* 27 April 2014. https://ocoy.org/the-5-kinds-of-modifications-of-the mind/

Adams, A. (2020). *Letters to Jonathan.* Self-Published by AndyHey Adams.

Admin. "The Seven Chakras for Beginners." *Hands on Health Sheffield.* January 27, 2020. http://www.handsonhealthsheffield.com/holistic_massage/the-seven-chakras-for-beginners/

Amodeo, J. *The Authentic Heart: An Eightfold Path to Midlife Love.* Hoboken, NJ: Wiley, 2001.

Angerame, L.D. "The Kleshas: Five Obstacles to Awareness." *Embodied Philosophy,* Issue 1. April 9, 2017. https://www.embodiedphilosophy.com/the-kleshas-five-obstacles-to-awareness-2/

Āraṇya, H. *Yoga Philosophy of Patañjali.* Albany, NY: State University of New York Press, 1983.

Avery, H. "108: Yoga's Sacred Number. *Wanderlust.* https://wanderlust.com/journal/108-yogas-sacred-number/

Bailey, G. and Mabbett, I. *The Sociology of Early Buddhism.* Cambridge, UK: Cambridge University Press, 2003.

Bajpai, R. S. *The Splendours and Dimensions of Yoga.* New Delhi: Motilal Banarsidass, 2002.

Bhadauria, A.S. Boost Thyself with Surya Namaskar. *Boost Thyself.*
December 29, 2017.
http://boostthyself.com/boost-thyself-with-surya-namaskar/

Bikram Yoga Asanas Chart. *Lewisberg District UMC.* n.d.
https://camaca.imaspmedia.com/bikram-yoga-asanas-chart/

"Breathing." *Joyful Garden Sangha.*
https://www.joyfulgarden.sg/mindfulness/

Bryant. E. "The Yoga Sūtras of Patañjali." *Internet Encyclopedia of Philosophy.*
https://iep.utm.edu/Yoga/

Bryant, E.F. *The Yoga Sūtras of Patañjali: A New Edition, Translation and Commentary.* New York: North Point Press, 2009.

Campbell, J. *Campbell and the Power of Myth with Bill Moyers.*
(B.S. Flowers, Ed.). New York, NY: Doubleday & Co, 1988.

Chödrön, P. *Start Where You Are: A Guide to Compassionate Living.*
Berkeley, CA: Shambala, 2018.

Chopra, D. *The Seven Spiritual Laws of Success.* 1994.
https://taxuna.files.wordpress.com/2015/11/deepak-chopra-the-7-laws-of-success.pdf

Chopra, D. "The Gap." *Deepak Chopra.* October 18, 2014.
https://www.deepakchopra.com/articles/the-gap/

Chopra, D. "Progress in the Gap." *Deepak Chopra.* May 12, 2020.
https://www.deepakchopra.com/articles/progress-in-the-gap/

Clarke, P.B. *New Religions in Global Perspective.* Oxfordshire, UK:
Routledge, 2006.

Daniélou, A. *Yoga: Mastering the Secrets of Matter and the Universe.*
Rochester, VT: Inner Traditions, 1991.

Desmarais, M.M. *Changing Minds: Mind, Consciousness and Identity in Patañjali's Yoga-Sūtra and Cognitive Neuroscience.* New Delhi: Motilal Banarsidass, 2008.

Devananda, S.V. *The Complete Illustrated Book of Yoga.* New York, NY: Three Rivers Press, 1995.

Dhand, A. "The dharma of ethics, the ethics of dharma: Quizzing the ideals of Hinduism." *Journal of Religious Ethics*, 30(3), 2002.

Dobrin, A. "Your Memory Isn't What You Think It Is." *Psychology Today*. July 16, 2013. https://www.psychologytoday.com/ca/blog/am-i-right/201307/your-memory-isnt-what-you-think-it-is

Doyle, L. *The Surrendered Wife: A Practical Guide for Finding Intimacy, Passion, and Peace with a Man*. New York, NY: Touchstone, 2001.

Dutt, H. *Immortal Speeches: New Delhi*. London, UK: Unicorn Books, 2005.

Edo & Jo—Topic. "Om Gam Ganapataye Namaha." YouTube video. 9:28. October 28, 2016. https://www.youtube.com/watch?v=F6BcPj42bUg

Edwards, H. and Smith, J.L. *My Secret Sister*. New York, NY: Pan Macmillan, 2013.

Edwards, M. "Stop Stretching Your Hamstrings!" *Huff Post*. March 18, 2017. Updated March 22, 2017. https://www.huffpost.com/entry/stop-stretching-your-hamstrings_b_58cdb802e4b0e0d348b34421

Eichenseer, M. "The Life Hack You Can Take Anywhere: Breathing." *Medium*. June 28, 2016. https://mikenseer.medium.com/the-life-hack-you-can-take-anywhere-breathing-20f0627d0f73

Feynman, R. *The Feynman Lectures on Physics, Volume 1*. Boston, MA: Addison Wesley, 1970. Chapter 4: "Conservation of Energy." https://www.feynmanlectures.caltech.edu/I_04.html

Garrigues, D. "84,000 postures and Krishnamacharya." *David Garrigues*. 2021. https://davidgarrigues.com/writings/84000-postures-and-krishnamacharya

Hewitt, J. *The Complete Yoga Book*. New York, NY: Schocken. 1990.

Iyengar, B.K.S. *Light on the Yoga Sūtras of Patañjali*. New York, NY: HarperCollins, 1993.

Jacuzzi, M. "Patañjali's Conception of the Mind." *Seven Winds Yoga & Jyotish*. 2005. http://www.sevenwindsYoga.com/writing/articles/Patañjali-s-conception-of-the-mind

K. Keegan, "Sutra 2.1: The Basics of Spiritual Discipline and Intro to Book 2" *No Big Secret Yoga & Astrology,* April 30, 2015.
http://no-bsyoga.com/keeganlife/2015/04/sutra-21.html

Kowalski, K. "What is Transcendence? The True Top of Maslow's Hierarchy of Needs." *Sloww.* https://www.sloww.co/transcendence-maslow/

Kurtus, R. "Four Noble Truths of Buddhism." *School for Champions.* October 6, 2018. https://www.school-for-champions.com/religion/buddhism_four_noble_truths.htm#.X_4qORNKiqA

Larson, C.D. *Your Forces and How to Use Them.* Eastford, CT: Martino Fine Books, 2012.

Lasater, J. "Beginning the Journey." *Yoga Journal,* Issue 6. 1998.

Lochtefeld, J.G. "Yama (2)." *The Illustrated Encyclopedia of Hinduism,* Vol. 2: N–Z. New York, NY: Rosen Publishing, 2000.

Long, J. *Jainism: An Introduction.* London, UK: IB Tauris, 2009.

Maslow, A.H. *The Farther Reaches of Human Nature.* New York, NY: Penguin Books, 1971.

Maxwell, J.C. *The Difference Maker.* New York, NY: HarperCollins Leadership, 2006.

McLeod, S. "Maslow's Hierarchy of Needs." *Simply Psychology.* December 29, 2020. https://www.simplypsychology.org/maslow.html

Messerly, J.G. "Summary of Maslow on Self-Transcendence." *Reason and Meaning.* January 18, 2017. https://reasonandmeaning.com/2017/01/18/summary-of-maslow-on-self-transcendence/

Mill, J.S. *Utilitarianism,* Chapter 2. 1863.
https://www.utilitarianism.com/mill2.htm

Nikam, N.A. Gandhi's Philosophy. *The Review of Metaphysics,* Vol. 7(4). 1954.

Nonya Business. "The Best First Date." YouTube video. 2:29. June 13, 2014.
https://www.youtube.com/watch?v=GiOJuIPl8vE

"Om Gam Ganapataye Namaha." *Yogapedia.* May 26, 2020.
https://www.Yogapedia.com/definition/9023/om-gam-ganapataye-namaha.

O'Toole, G. "With Great Power Comes Great Responsibility." *Quote Investigator*. July 23, 2015. Updated July 24, 2015. https://quoteinvestigator.com/2015/07/23/great-power/.

Pearce, J.C. *The Biology of Transcendence: A Blueprint of the Human Spirit*. New York, NY: Simon and Shuster, 2004.

Perrotta, M. "Controlling Your Mind by Controlling Your Breath." *The Startup*. June 10, 2020. https://medium.com/swlh/neuroscience-of-breath-63c32604be22

Phillips, S.H. *Yoga, Karma, and Rebirth: A Brief History and Philosophy*. New York, NY: Columbia University Press, 2013.

Planck, M. *Treatise on Thermodynamics* (3rd Ed., A. Ogg, Trans.). London: Longmans, Green & Co, 1927.

Prabhavananda, S. "Patañjali Yoga Sūtras." *Sri Ramakrishna Math*. 1953. https://estudantedavedanta.net/Yoga-Aphorisms-of-Patañjali.pdf

Radhakrishnan, S. and Moore, C.A. *A Source Book in Indian Philosophy*. Princeton, NJ: Princeton University Press, 1989.

Raghupathi, K.V. *Yoga for Peace*. India: Abhinav Publications, 2007.

Ramamurti, M. *Fundamentals of Yoga*. (2nd Ed.). New York: Baba Bhagavandas Publication Trust, 2002.

Rumi, J. A-D. *The Essential Rumi*. Trans. Coleman Barks. NJ: Castle Books, 1997.

Salzberg, S. *Lovingkindness: The Revolutionary Art of Happiness*. Berkeley, CA: Shambala, 1995.

Sayadaw, M. *Brahmavihara Dhamma* (Part II). 1983. http://www.buddhanet.net/brahmaviharas/bvd020.htm.

Scharfe, H. "Education in India." *Handbook of Oriental Studies, Volume 2: South Asia*. The Netherlands: Brill, 2002.

"Sisters and Brothers of America": Full text of Swami Vivekananda's historic speech in 1893. *DNA India*. https://www.dnaindia.com/india/report-telling-the-world-about-hinduism-full-text-of-swami-vivekananda-s-historic-speech-in-1893-2164870

Sovik, R. and Ravizza, D. "Self-Study: Nostril Dominance." *Yoga International.* https://Yogainternational.com/article/view/self-study-nostril-dominance

Sullivan, H.P. "Isvara." *Encyclopedia of Religion.* (M. Eliade, Ed.). New York: MacMillan Publishing, 1987.

Sterbenz, C. "12 Famous Quotes That Always Get Misattributed." *Business Insider.* 7 October 2013. https://www.businessinsider.com/misattributed-quotes-2013-10#:~:text=AP%20Photo%20We've%20all,He%20never%20said%20it

Swami, O. "The Four Pillars of Sādhanā." *Om Swami.* December 22, 2011. https://os.me/the-four-pillars-of-sadhana/

Thomas, K. "Lost Generation Part 5: Statistics on father-deprived children." *Canadian Association for Equality.* November 25, 2014. https://equalitycanada.com/lost-generation-part-5-statistics-on-father-deprived-children/

Thoughts, T. *Tears of a Teenage Mother.* Bloomington, IN: AuthorHouse, 2012.

Tigunait, P.R. Yoga Sūtra 1.6-1.7 Translation and Commentary. 2021. *Yoga International.* https://Yogainternational.com/article/view/Yoga-Sūtra-1-6-1-7-translation-and-commentary

University of North Carolina. "Brief meditative exercise helps cognition." *Science Daily*, April 19, 2010. www.sciencedaily.com/releases/2010/04/100414184220.htm

van Eijck, J. "Logic, Rationality, and Common Sense (3)." *Vaneijck.org.* June 14, 2017. http://vaneijck.org/posts/2017-06-14-commonsense.html

Vasudev, J. "The What & Why of Sādhanā." *Official Website of Sadhguru, Isha Foundation.* December 6, 2012. https://isha.sadhguru.org/ca/en/wisdom/article/the-what-why-of-sadhana

Vivekananda, S. *The Complete Works of Swami Vivekananda, Volume I: Addresses at The Parliament of Religions, Karma-Yoga, Raja-Yoga, Lectures and Discourses.* New York: Discovery, 2017.

White, D.G. *The Yoga Sūtra of Patañjali: A Biography*. Princeton, NJ: Princeton University Press, 2014.

Wood, J. *The Yoga System of Patañjali*. Cambridge, MA: Harvard University Press, 1914. https://archive.org/stream/Yogasystemofpata00wooduoft#page/178/mode/2up

Woolf, V. *The Moment and Other Essays*. Project Gutenberg Australia, 1947. http://gutenberg.net.au/ebooks15/1500221h.html

Yamamoto, K. *The Mahayana Mahaparinirvana Sūtra*. Translated into English from Dharmakshema's Chinese version in Taisho Tripitaka, Vol. 12, No. 374. 1973. https://www.nirvanaSūtra.net/convenient/Mahaparinirvana_Sūtra_Yamamoto.pdf

Yoga Association of Seychelles *Branches of Yoga*. http://Yogaassociationofseychelles.weebly.com/about-Yoga.html

Yoga Sūtra Study. YSP-Sūtras 1.01-1.20. Chapter 1: "Samadhi Pada." *Yoga Sūtra Study: Path to Enlightenment*. 2021. https://YogaSūtrastudy.info/Yoga-Sūtra-translations/ysp-Sūtras1-01-1-20/

Zukav, G. *The Seat of the Soul: 25th Anniversary Edition*. New York, NY: Simon and Schuster, 2007.

CPSIA information can be obtained
at www.ICGtesting.com
Printed in the USA
BVHW020041181022
649620BV00001B/1